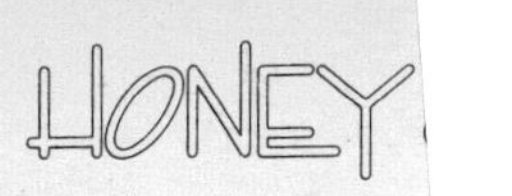

Examines the medical evide
a natural foo

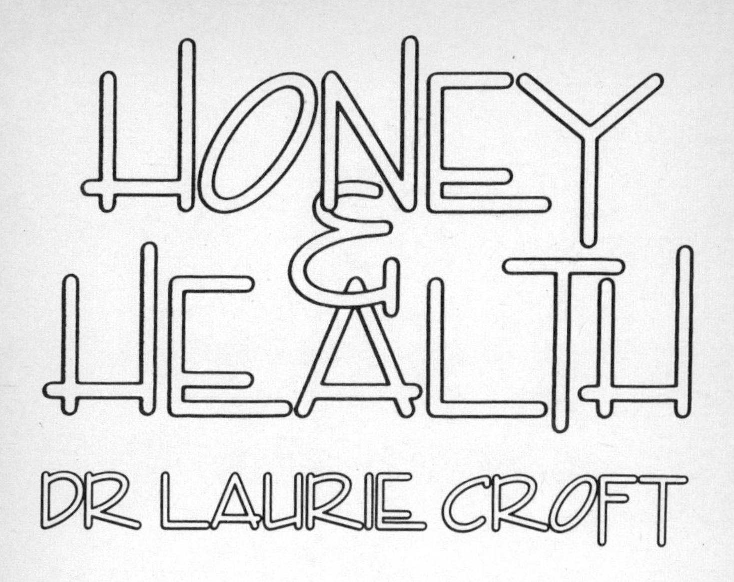

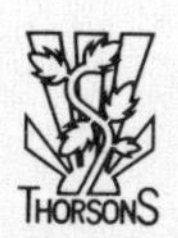

THORSONS PUBLISHING GROUP
Wellingborough, Northamptonshire

Rochester, Vermont

First published May 1987

British Library Cataloguing in Publication Data

Croft, Laurie
Honey and health.
1. Honey — Therapeutic use
I. Title
615.8'54 RM666.H55

ISBN 0-7225-1389-5

Printed and bound in Great Britain

Contents

THE AUTHOR

Dr Laurie Croft graduated with First Class honours from the University of Nottingham in 1965. For his doctorate he carried out research on the tuberculostatic antibiotics viomycin and capreomycin. From 1968 until 1973 he was a member of staff of the Medical School of the University of Oxford, where he carried out research into the causes of cataract. Since 1973 he has been a lecturer in the University of Salford and has continued research into a number of medical problems, including, ageing and abnormal haemoglobins. Since 1980 he has done novel research on honey, covering both analytical and medical aspects, and has become well known as a lecturer on this subject throughout the country.

Preface

It is unfortunate that most serious researchers tend to steer well clear of alternative medicine. Clearly there is some loss of credibility even to be vaguely associated with it. However, what many people fail to realise is that alternative medicine, or rather as I see it, natural medicine, is a very broad and heterogeneous area. Indeed, there are many practices that are frankly fraudulent, and others that are foolishly harmless. But, conventional medicine is not exactly faultless. There is good and bad in most things and it is surely wrong to condemn all forms of natural medicine outright. There are areas that are useful, and I believe honey, as a natural medicine, is one of them.

I am not the first to hold this view. Even in recent times a number of serious books have appeared promulgating the possible role of honey in medicine. The approach I have adopted is, however, rather different in that I have attempted to understand and explain the possible mechanisms that might exist for the curative properties of honey. Furthermore, I have attempted to do this without the necessity of reciting unconvincing and vague anecdotes that one usually finds in a book of this type.

Laurie Croft

CHAPTER 1

Honey: an Ancient Medicine

The use of honey in the treatment of internal and external maladies must be much older than the history of medicine itself. How did early man come to choose honey for this purpose? We know for instance that many animals instinctively eat what is good for them. Man also has powerful instinctive impulses to eat certain foods at particular times. It is therefore likely that primitive man in his search for curative natural substances in his environment must have discovered honey at an early stage and become convinced of its supreme curative value. How else can we account for the almost universal belief in the medical value of honey?

Today, if we look at the chemical analysis of honey we see that although much has been found out about its composition we, as yet, cannot account for its medical attributes. Accordingly many scientists and doctors have only too readily accepted the view that the whole thing is a myth. It is less easy in our technological age to accept, or even contemplate, the alternative. Let us look at the facts before accepting either version.

It is true that the major components of honey have now been identified and characterized and that none of them can explain many of its supposed medical applications. However there are still a great many minor constituents that have not yet been characterized. Could possibly one, or two, of these substances have the biological properties that might account for the legendary medical value of honey? The alternative is to dismiss all the historical evidence. Can we say that all this evidence, gained not in any laboratory, but from generations of human experience, is all supposition? This is the theme that I hope to develop in the subsequent chapters of this small book, but to begin with we will take a glimpse at some of the historical evidence.

Ancient Egypt

The earliest references to the medical uses of honey appear in ancient Egyptian texts. The first known medical text is the Kahun papyrus which appeared in the Middle Kingdom around 2000 BC. Over a period of about 1000 years many medical texts appeared, but it is the earlier ones that are most significant. Many of the later ones become ill-defined and tend to become bogged down with such things as witchcraft. In total if they were to be translated and typed on A4 paper they would amount to about 500 pages. In essence they consist of many short statements and prescriptions along with short descriptions of common diseases.

In the most famous one the so-called 'Smith' papyrus, we discover that honey, or 'Byt', is symbolized in hieroglyphics as a bee and is mentioned about 500 times out of a total of 900 prescriptions.

In general, Egyptian remedies tend to include long lists of possible substitutes such as egg white, or goat's milk, and so on. Often these possible alternatives are reinforced with comments like: 'excellent' . . . 'good' . . . 'very effective'. But, whenever honey is mentioned it is with complete bluntness and no superlatives are given. This would be much the same way as we would mention penicillin today, and leads us to assume that the author of the document was really confident in the effectiveness of honey, and knew without any doubt that it really did work.

The standard wound salve in the 'Smith' papyrus is a mixture of grease and honey. This is also the case in the 'Ebers' papyrus which, at twenty metres in length, is the longest manuscript. In this papyrus we find a remedy for ear trouble as grease (two-thirds) and honey (one-third).

The grease, or 'mrht' as it is called, was anything from vegetable oil, snake grease, beef fat, to butter. Today we have many ointments that have a lanolin base, which is not so very different from ox grease, or for that matter snake fat!

Although the proportion of honey to grease is found in the 'Ebers' manuscript, in other instances the ratios are omitted and might indicate that they were well known and widely used.

It is easy to dismiss all this as myth, but before one does, it is worth mentioning that many widespread traditional cures for many common complaints have been substantiated by modern science. For example, we know that one cause of night blindness, is due to vitamin A deficiency. The traditional cure for this is actually mentioned in the 'Ebers' papyrus as liver, which we now know is rich in vitamin A.

The society that was able to construct the great pyramids had sufficient skills and intelligence to interpret and learn from empirical observations as to how best to effectively treat many of the common diseases. As honey was so universally employed in their system of medicine it might indicate that our present assumption that honey is simply a pleasant item of food could be a serious devaluation.

Ancient India

Another old civilization that has put significant value on the use of honey in medicine is that of ancient India. Around 1500 BC the original dark-skinned inhabitants of India were overrun by lighter-skinned people known as the Aryans. Until quite recently beekeeping was carried on in Cashmere in much the same way as it was by the original Aryan peoples. As each house was built, space would be left in the walls in which hives would be kept. The wall cavities would be carefully lined with a mixture of mortar, clay and chopped straw. The inner end would be closed with a large flat tile. Up to a dozen hives would be kept in each house. At the end of the season the father of the household would collect the honey. Smoke would be blown into the cavity from a smouldering wisp of straw in order to subjugate the bees and the honeycombs removed. The bees were not destroyed and so the same colonies of bees could be used in the following seasons.

The language of the Aryans had originated from the same source as that of classical Greece and Rome. From it developed Sanskrit which became the language of the elite. Aryan literature is also in Sanskrit. In their four sacred books, known as the Vedas, we find references to the use of honey in their system of medicine. The fourth Veda is the *Atharva Veda* and contains the Hindu system of medicine known as 'Ayurveda'. Ayurveda medicine is based essentially on two treatises. One by Charaka, the so-called 'Charaka Samhita' is entirely medical. The other by Sushruta the 'Sushruta Samhita' is mainly surgical. It is not possible to date these treatises with any degree of accuracy, but it is generally thought that they are at least 3000 years old. Both consist of collections of treatments for common complaints. Sushruta, being a surgeon, describes the extensive use of honey in the management of wounds. Eight types of honey are mentioned and each had specific medical uses and properties. Some honeys were recommended for treating asthma, whereas others were thought best for curing difficult skin diseases. It is interesting that an ointment made of honey and butter was universally employed in Ayurvedic surgery and resembled the wound salve of ancient Egypt.

In general, the Ayurvedic manuscripts give great prominence to the widespread use of honey and conclude that human life may be prolonged if honey is a significant part of the diet.

Before we dismiss these sentiments it is well to reflect on the many authenticated reports of centenarians who have been beekeepers, or users of honey as a substantial part of their diet. Professor N. N. Godbole, a famous Indian scientist who has researched the use of honey in Ayurvedic medicine has written: 'although the chemical constituents of honey were hardly known, yet the practical application and pharmacopoeia of honey were well studied, fully understood and intelligently applied and administered.'

Islamic Medicine

The Islamic people have a deep respect for the medical virtues of honey. The prophet Muhammed, who founded the religion, lived from AD 571 to AD 632. In the Islamic holy book, the *Koran*, or *Al-Quraan*, there is a complete chapter on the bee entitled 'Sura-Alnahal'. In this we read: 'And the Lord inspired the bee. . . . There cometh from their bellies a drink diverse of hues, where is healing for mankind. Lo! herein is indeed a portent for people who reflect.' This explicit reference to the medical importance of honey has been proved throughout the ages by many of the followers of Islam. Even today Islamic people follow Muhammed in firmly believing that honey is natural medicine of tremendous value.

Ancient Greece and Rome

In ancient Greece honey was considered to be a valuable gift of nature. Aristotle, in the fourth century BC wrote at great length about honey, as did Homer in the *Iliad* and the *Odyssey*. In the third century AD Athenaeus informs us that the followers of Pythagoras ate honey daily and attributed their long lives to this habit.

Pliny, the Elder, who lived from AD 23 until his sudden death at Pompeii in AD 79, wrote that for long life and good health honey should be eaten daily. This was no idle speculation but was based on his own surveys carried out during his extensive travelling. During these journeys he witnessed at first hand many communities of long-lived people that shared a common factor, namely, the regular consumption of honey.

Hippocrates, the father of medicine, was also an ardent advocate of the use of honey. He claimed that it was invaluable in the management of wounds and ulcers, and also recommended it for respiratory disorders and skin complaints. Dioscorides, the Greek physician of the first century AD, renowned for his famous work *Materia Medica*, put much emphasis on the therapeutic use of honey.

China

In ancient China honey was an important natural medicine. As the sugar cane plant was native to China, honey was not traditionally employed as a sweetener, but solely as a medicine. It was consequently greatly prized and in one ancient manuscript it was described as the 'drug of immortality'. Even to this day honey has a significant role in the traditional medicine of China.

Russia

Beekeeping has always been important to the Russian economy and society. In the old traditional medicine of this country, the village folk physician relied on honey as a universal remedy. These people had received their training from life and it is difficult to accept that they would have relied on honey as much as they did if they had not seen many effective cures. Thus in many of the old Russian medical manuscripts, and in folk songs and epic poems, we find that honey is continually lauded as a wonderful medicine. Would they have developed this tradition if honey was not effective? I think not.

Many people now recognise that folk medicine has done much to advance scientific medicine, many drugs, for example, have had their origin in popular medicine — digitalis, cocaine, quinine and atropine to name just a few. Even penicillin, in the form of its parent mould, was in use in popular medicine, long before its scientific discovery. If we look carefully today we find that in general the drugs that are most useful to man, in terms of effectiveness and least side effects, have been largely derived from observations taken from folk medicine. The greatest advance in modern medicine, namely our understanding of the immune system and the consequent development of vaccines and so on, had its origin in folk medicine.

During the last two hundred years our scientific knowledge has advanced by leaps and bounds. Hence, in dealing with improbable statements which have come down to us from classical or mediaeval times, we tend to be too ready to dismiss them as myths and superstitions, instead of seeking for the substratum of truth that often underlies them. I hope in this small book to look at the use of honey in medicine, to dust away some of the myth and see what possible truth there is beneath.

CHAPTER 2

Honey: a Natural Food

Man has only two wholly natural foods, one is milk and the other is honey. Since antiquity both of these substances have been closely associated. It is probable that primitive man found that he could maintain full health and strength on these two materials alone. In time they became elevated to a high position of importance. Eventually this turned to reverence. We therefore find in several early cultures that both milk and honey are used as frequent offerings to their respective gods.

Today we are able to appreciate how such a combination may provide all the necessary nutritional requirements. Milk, for example, is rich in protein and honey in carbohydrate; and between the two there are sufficient trace minerals and vitamins. Furthermore, it has been proved by experiment that man can survive indefinitely on this very simple diet.

At what stage in man's evolution did he recognize the beneficial properties of honey? We cannot know. Possibly it may have been entirely instinctive. Many lower animals seek out the bee for its honey. The starling, for example, will catch a bee and peck out its honey-containing stomach. In literature there are several accounts of country children catching bees for the same purpose. Oliver Goldsmith in his *Animated Nature* wrote:

> As for the honey, it is extracted from that part of the flower called the nectareum. From the mouth this delicious fluid passes into the gullet: and then into the first stomach, or honey-bag, which when filled appears like an oblong bladder. Children, that live in country places, are well acquainted with this bladder: and destroy many bees to come at their store of honey.

And Gilbert White, in his *Natural History of Selborne*, gave a detailed account of a boy who hunted bees on account of their honey-sacs.

We know very little about the diet of early man. Much has to be based on assumption and supposition, however we can be almost certain that honey played a significant role. The legacy today is found in the universal acclaim given to honey by all races and cultures.

The earliest direct evidence of man's interest in honey is to be found in the famous Stone-Age cave paintings in Southern Spain. One in the Arâna cave near Bicorp, Valencia, illustrates a honey gatherer raiding a bees' nest. The man's approach is almost exactly the same as that described by Alfred Wallace (1823–1913) in his account of how the natives in Timor would ascend the trunks of lofty forest trees in their search for honeycombs.

Early man was therefore a bee-hunter, rather than a bee-keeper. Presumably there existed such an abundance of wild bee colonies, in rocks and in trees, that there was ample honey for the taking. There are many parts of the world where such natural abundances of wild bees' nests have been described. For example, on the precipitous slopes of the Teesta valley in India, tradition has it that there existed enormous natural colonies of bees. On the plain of Troy, the Bali-dagh, or 'Honey Mount' is so named on account of the numerous wild bees that live in caves on the precipitous south side. Israel, also, must have been such a place. For in the Bible we find many descriptions and allusions to both bees and honey, but nothing about the keeping of bees.

Biblical References

We can learn much about the early use of honey in man's diet from Biblical references. However, care is needed in their interpretation as several Hebrew words have been translated in our Bible as 'honey' but do not in fact refer to 'bee-honey'. This is also seen in the writings of Flavius Josephus, in particular, in his *Jewish Antiquities*, he mentions the excellence of the honey found in the locality of Jericho, and mentions one as 'bee-honey' and the other as 'vegetable-honey'. This being a syrup made from pressed dates.

Bee-honey, however, is clearly referred to in the first book of Samuel. In chapter fourteen we read of Jonathan entering a forest on Mount Ephraim and finding honey literally flowing from the trees and spilling on the ground. This must have been bee-honey for although it is exceptional for bees to allow honey to overflow from the honeycombs, it does occasionally occur, particularly during a heavy nectar flow, as any beekeeper will verify. Indeed, travellers to Israel in more recent times have recorded seeing enormous honeycombs hanging from trees with honey actually dripping from them.

Honey was an abundant and widely-used food in Palestine, thus we read in Ezekiel 16:13 'thou didst eat fine flour and honey. . .' But beekeeping does not seem to have been practised. The inhabitants of Palestine during the period covered by the Old Testament appeared to have been honey-hunters rather than beekeepers. Thus we read in Proverbs 25:16 'Hast thou *found* honey?' In the countryside bees would frequently build nests in the side of cliffs and rocks, and so we read in Deuteronomy 32:13 'he made him to suck honey out of the rock. . .' and in Psalm 81:16, 'He should have fed them also with the finest of the wheat: and with honey out of the rock. . .'

There is also the well-known, and much debated account of Samson in the book of Judges 14:8–9; 'he turned aside to see the carcase of the lion: and behold there was a swarm of bees and honey in the carcase of the lion. And he took thereof in his hands and went on eating . . .'

In the New Testament we read in Matthew's Gospel that John the Baptist 'had his raiment of camel's hair, and a leathern girdle about his loins: and his meat was locusts and wild honey' (3:4).

Ancient Egypt

Thus from the Biblical record we find that in Palestine there existed places abundant in wild honey. In these areas the actual keeping of bees would be unnecessary. We may assume therefore that early man would not have evolved a system of bee husbandry until he was forced to do so on account of a local shortage of honey. This situation could have arisen as a consequence of climatic change, however, as the honey-bee is remarkably adaptable to climate this seems unlikely. It is much more likely that a decrease in bee colonies would have been brought about by localised disease. We know today that there are parts of the world where certain honey-bee diseases are endemic. In these areas the number of wild bee colonies would be severely reduced. This may have forced early man to devise a way of maintaining bees in a semi-domesticated manner. Such a situation may have existed in ancient Egypt, for we find the earliest extant records of beekeeping in drawings from this period. For example, on a relief in the Fifth-Dynasty temple of Niweserre at Abusir, built around 2500 BC, there are scenes depicting early beekeeping. The hives appear as cylindrical pipes piled up in horizontal rows. Each hollow tube, made of sun-baked mud, appears to be about four feet in length and about eight inches in diameter. The pipes are laid together in a pile protected from the heat of the sun by a coating of mud or, in some cases, branches of trees. Similar hives remain the traditional hive in many parts of the Middle East to this day.

In ancient Egypt honey was widely used as part of the diet. In the tomb of Rekhara of the Eighteenth Dynasty built around 1500 BC, there are drawings showing men baking honey cakes. We also know from surviving records that Rameses III made a gift of 7050 jars of honey to a foreign king.

The ancient Egyptians also engaged in migratory beekeeping, much as beekeepers on the Nile have done in more recent times. Hives were moved along the Nile on large rafts so as to keep pace with the changing blossoms. On reaching Cairo the honey was extracted and sold. A document has recently been discovered, dating from about 250 BC, which appears to be a petition from beekeepers who are pleading to an official called Zenon, for the supply of donkeys needed to tow the rafts to a new area.

Honey as a food preservative

In other ancient cultures honey has also played a significant role. In India one of the purificatory ceremonies of the Hindus was that of placing honey in the mouth of a new-born male child. The tradition of feeding infants honey seems particularly widespread. In the book of Isaiah 7:14, 15 we read: 'Behold, a virgin shall conceive, and bear a son, and shall call his name Immanuel. Butter and honey shall he eat . . .' Solomon, also wrote: 'my son, eat thou honey, because it is good . . .' It is easy to see how this tradition evolved. There are few foods that may be safely given to small infants without risking infection. Honey, being completely sterile, was one considered safe to be given infants.*

Another old Hindu tradition was the making a gift of honey and butter to a welcomed guest, or bridegroom. Such a combination of honey and butter might seem unlikely, and not appeal to our palates today, but it was a traditional dish in many Eastern countries. The nineteenth century

*There has been recent concern in the United States over the advisability of feeding honey to young infants (cf. S. S. Arnon, *Ann. Rev. Med.*, (1980) *31*, p. 541-560). American honey companies have responded by warning parents not to feed honey to infants less than twelve months old. As, at the time of writing, the position in Britain is still unclear, it would be prudent to follow the American advice and not to feed honey to very young infants.

traveller D'Arvieux described in his *Memoirs* (iii, 209) this customary dish:

> One of their chief breakfasts is cream or fresh butter mixed with honey : these do not seem to suit very well together : but experience teaches that this is no bad mixture nor disagreeable in its taste if one is ever so little accustomed to it.

Captain Charles Irby in his book *Travels in Egypt, Nubia, Syria and Asia Minor* writes of the same custom: 'They gave us honey and butter together with bread to dip in Narsah desiring one of his men to mix it for us. The Arab stirred it with his fingers, showed his dexterity at consuming as well as mixing.' There are also many Biblical references to this dish, as in Isaiah 7:22; . . . for butter and honey shall every one eat that is left in the land.' and, 2 Samuel 17:27–29;

> And it came to pass when David was come to Mahanaim, that Shobi the son of Nahash of Rabbah of the children of Ammon . . . Brought beds and basons, and earthen vessels, and wheat and barley, and flour, and parched corn, and beans, and lentils, and parched pulse, and honey, and butter . . . for David, and for the people that were with him, to eat.

One can appreciate that for nomadic people, particularly those living in a hot climate, mixing honey with butter would have been a means of preserving the latter. Honey therefore was not only important as a food, but as a food preservative. Along with salt, honey was probably one of the first natural food preservatives. Indeed we find today that in Eastern countries honey is widely used in the preservation of fresh fruit. This application would have added greater value to honey as a commodity, so in the book of Jeremiah 41:8 we find honey referred to as a 'treasure', thus: 'But ten men were found among them that said unto Ishmael, slay us not: for we have *treasures* in the field, of wheat, and of barley, and of oil, and of honey. So he forebare and slew them not . . .'

Ancient Greece and Rome

Throughout antiquity honey was used in religious ceremonies. The ancient people of Peru offered honey to their sun-god. In ancient Greece a honey cake was the food of the fabled serpent-guardian of the Acropolis. From earliest times honey, milk and wine formed the triple offering to the dead. In the eleventh book of the *Odyssey*, which outlines Odysseus' visit to the nether world, the author describes the ritual with its triple libation of honey mixed with milk, sweet wine and water.

Greek honey has been renowned throughout history for its unique quality. One reason for this is that the Athenian beekeepers rarely ever used smoke to subjugate the bees while harvesting the honey. Smoke is usually used today for this purpose and has been used since the Stone Age. The Greek beekeepers chose not to use smoke and so their honey was of greater purity and had enhanced flavour. In particular, the honey collected from the region of Mount Hymettus, which in the main was from wild thyme, had a special reputation. And that of Attica was already famous in the time of Solon, around 594 BC.

In Roman times honey was widely used both in the diet and as a food preservative. Considerable insight as to its widespread use is to be found in the first chapter of *The Roman Cookery Book* written by Coelius Apicius. Each villa would have an enclosure set apart for the beehives which were tended by a slave known as the 'mellarius'. Some indication as to the relative importance of beekeeping in Roman agriculture is gained from the fact that Virgil (70–19 BC) devotes one whole book, out of a total of four, of his *Georgics* or *Art of Husbandry* entirely to the art of beekeeping. Virgil also describes how honey is harvested and used. He mentions its use to improve the quality of poor wine thus:

You'll strain sweet honey, sweet and clear enough.
To tame the bitter flavour of the wine.

Mead

This practice of adding honey to poor quality wines seems to have been widely adopted. 'Mulsum' is the usual name given to wine which has had honey added. In Scotland there is a liquor known as 'Athole Brose' which is prepared from equal parts of heather honey and whisky.

Mead is, however, the usual alcoholic drink prepared from honey. But, as honey is lacking in certain nutrients it is not particularly easy to ferment. This may have led many individuals to rather add the honey to an already fermented drink. In Chaucer's time a beverage known as 'Piment' or 'Pyment' was a wine to which honey had been added. Similarly 'Bracket' was an ale which was sweetened with honey. In fact, until quite recently, it was possible to buy, in some parts of Northern England, a local beer known as 'honey beer'.

For the ancient British, ordinary mead was the main alcoholic drink. Although we know very little about beekeeping at that time we may assume, from the fact that several of the early Roman writers called Britain the 'Isle of Honey', that beekeeping was widely practised. In addition, as the countryside was mainly forested, there would have been an abundance of wild bee colonies. These bees would have been our native black bees, a strain of bee notable for its hardiness and industry. Accordingly we can assume that great harvests of honey were obtained by the early British beekepers.

Mead would normally be prepared from the honeycombs after the honey had been drained off. The combs would be immersed in water and left to ferment. This would result in the traditional mead. With time, however, many variations were introduced. Details of some of these have survived in ancient writings. 'Morat' for example, was prepared from fermented mulberry juice and honey. 'Metheglin', or as it was sometimes known 'hydromel' was a dry mead to which herbs and spices had been added. 'Sackmead' was a traditionally-prepared mead to which hops had been added. Similar, related, alcoholic beverages occur in other honey-rich countries. In Russia, for example, a famous mead known as 'Lipetz' has been prepared for many centuries past from the delicious lime honey which is abundant in that country.

Thus we may conclude that sometime in the distant past man discovered that honey was a delicious and nutritional food, that required no processing, or preparation. He must have concluded that as it never appeared to go 'bad' then it was safe to feed to infants. Furthermore as it never appeared to deteriorate then this might have suggested to him that it could be used to prevent other foods from going off. In addition to all this he must have discovered at a very early stage that it could be the basis of an enjoyable beverage. It is not surprising, therefore, that to many of the ancient peoples, honey was seen to be a 'gift of the gods'.

CHAPTER 3

From Nectar to Honey

Nectar is a secretion of specific glands that are normally located in a flower at the base of the stamen. These glands are known as nectaries and are just visible to the naked eye. Although they may superficially appear to be merely holes in the plant tissue they are in fact much more complicated than they seem and act as sophisticated organs regulating the composition and flow of nectar. Although nectar is a secretion of fluid that is unwanted by the plant, it does have a secondary function in that it serves as an attractant for insects. One may presume that throughout the long process of plant evolution this process has developed as a means for assisting the plant to reproduce. For the insect, attracted by the nectar, unwittingly transfers pollen from one plant to another. Thus the whole intricate process appears to have been stage-managed to a high degree of perfection by the determinants of the evolutionary process.

The plant, however, by depending on the insect for such a vital role, is taking a considerable risk. Normally, plants prefer to deter insects. Many of them produce within their tissues substances that are highly toxic to insects. For example the insecticides, derris, pyrethrum and quassia are all derived from plant tissue. All amateur gardeners know that a very effective insecticide may be made from the nicotine in cigarette tobacco, again derived from the leaf of a plant. And a large section of the horticultural industry is concerned with finding ways of deterring insects from plants, so why are insects bad for plants? The answer is simple — because they carry disease.

All gardeners are well aware of how quickly disease may spread from one plant to another, and in the main, the agent which is responsible for this transference, is insects. It therefore seems an enigma that on the one hand plants go to such lengths to deter insects and yet at the same time depend upon them for the vital task of reproduction.

Such an arrangement could only have successfully evolved if the plant had within its attractant, namely the nectar, certain substances able to destroy, or at least neutralize, any disease organism brought there by an insect.

The organisms causing possible disease include bacteria, fungi and viruses. Thus one might expect to find within nectar antibacterial, antifungal and antiviral substances. But surely chemists have analysed nectar? Yes, much work has been published on the analysis of nectar, which shows it to be largely a solution of various sugars in water, together with a large number of minor components including amino acids, vitamins, proteins and enzymes. Antimicrobial substances would be expected to be present in very low concentration and so would not readily be identifiable. Although speculation in science is discouraged, a limited amount is legitimate, particularly if it has some basis in fact. Therefore let us go one step further in our argument and draw the conclusion that if these substances are present in nectar, then they would also be present in honey. In fact, as honey is a concentrated form of nectar they would be present at a much higher concentration. Could this account for the remarkable antibiotic properties of honey that have been recorded throughout history? This argument will be developed further in subsequent chapters, but before we do that, let us look at how the nectar is transformed into honey. To begin with let us examine its composition.

As already mentioned, the main constituents of nectar are various sugars. This is true also for honey. The precise type of sugar present in nectar depends largely upon the plant. However, environmental conditions, particularly temperature, humidity and water retention of the soil are also important. It is largely the quantity and type of sugar present in the nectar that ultimately determines the character and amount of honey produced. Nectars vary considerably in their flavour and sweetness. Plum nectar, for example, has a low concentration of sucrose; lime and clover have average amounts, whereas marjoram nectar has a very high concentration. Bees are very selective in the nectar they collect. They are able to identify which nectar is richest in sugar, and so collect that. Many novice beekeepers make the mistake of planting what they consider to be suitable flowers around their beehives only to watch in disappointment as their bees fly well away to collect nectar somewhere else.

The actual process of collecting nectar from the plant is as follows:

the bee, on arriving at a flower, will insert its proboscis into the nectary and suck. She will take as much nectar as possible and then fly on to another flower. In this way she gradually fills her honey-sac which might take up to an hour, and involve visiting about a hundred separate flowers. Under normal circumstances she will concentrate on one species of flower at a time.

A simple calculation may be performed to determine how much effort is involved in collecting enough nectar to produce one kilogram of honey. The honey-sac of an individual bee when full contains around 50 milligrams of nectar, which, on processing, produces about half as much honey. If we assume that the normal distance foraged is between one and two miles distant from the hive, then the bee will need to travel approximately 250,000 miles, to produce one kilogram of honey!

During the process of collecting the nectar the bee is continuously adding to it certain enzymes, in particular invertase. This enzyme causes the sucrose in the nectar to break down into glucose and fructose. On reaching the hive the returning honey-bee immediately regurgitates the nectar and passes it on to other house bees. These particular bees manipulate the nectar in their mouth parts adding to it more invertase and the amino acid proline. (What purpose the latter substance has is not known.) Eventually, after the nectar has been passed from house bee to house bee, it is deposited into an empty cell in the honeycomb. At the next stage in the process the water content of the partially-formed honey is slowly reduced by evaporation, which is enhanced by the general warmth of the hive and the activity of the house bees known as 'fanning'. This is a highly organized and concerted activity designed to create a flow of warm air over the combs.

When the water content of the honey reaches about eighteen per cent and each of the cells in the honeycomb filled completely with honey, they are then 'capped'. This involves sealing the cell with an airtight covering of beeswax. This seal prevents the honey absorbing any further moisture from the environment which would otherwise cause it to ferment. Finally the bee injects through the seal a small amount of its venom. This is further insurance against the honey decomposing.

Important chemical changes take place during the concentration of the nectar, due to the presence of enzymes previously added by the bee. In particular the enzyme invertase transforms the sucrose in the nectar into a mixture of glucose and fructose. In chemical terms sucrose may be looked upon as a compound of glucose and fructose. Invertase acts simply to split the larger sugar into two smaller ones. We can mimic this chemical reaction in the laboratory by heating a solution of sucrose with a dilute acid. In fact this is frequently accomplished in the kitchen when, for example, sugar is heated with chopped-up rhubarb. In this case the acids in the plant tissue are sufficiently strong enough to convert the sucrose into its component sugars, glucose and fructose.

Bees effect the same transformation with the enzyme invertase. The enzyme, however, is able to work at a much lower temperature and very much more quickly. Bees, apparently, have evolved this ability of employing this enzyme over many millions of years. Furthermore its use has important significance, for, by being able to convert sucrose into glucose and fructose, the bee is able to store within the honeycomb a much greater quantity of carbohydrate.

This may be illustrated by considering the simple manufacturing process of making soft-centre chocolates. These are made by a very simple process involving the enzyme invertase. A small quantity of this enzyme is mixed with sucrose, to which has been added an appropriate flavouring, and then cast into a suitable shape. When solid it is coated with chocolate and allowed to cool. During this process the enzyme invertase is slowly breaking down the sucrose. Eventually most of the sucrose will have been converted into glucose and fructose which are more soluble than the previously solid sucrose. The centre will now be semi-liquid.

Evolution has provided bees with the same enzyme so that they may store in their honeycomb a greater quantity of carbohydrate. But whereas man has been using invertase in the food industry for a matter of only a few decades, the bee has been carrying out the same process for the past 100 million years!

CHAPTER 4

What is Honey?

We have seen in the preceding chapter that honey is produced by bees from the nectar secreted by flowering plants. Let us now turn our attention to the composition of honey. There exists a common misunderstanding that honey is obtained from plants. This error is compounded by our common practice of calling a honey after a particular plant source. Thus we refer to 'lime' honey from lime trees, and 'heather' honey from heather and so on. What in fact we mean is that the honey is made by the bee from that particular plant nectar. As we have already discussed in the previous chapter, honey may be seen to have been 'manufactured' by the bees from nectar.

As a manufactured product it cannot be looked upon as a chemical compound but as a delicately balanced mixture of sugars and other substances dissolved in water. Analytical chemists have been studying honey for well over a century, and many of its components have been identified. Indeed, scientists have been so confident as to suppose that they could produce an entirely artificial honey. But despite their confidence this project has met with miserable failure.

Physical Aspects

Colour

Before we take a look at the various constituents it is appropriate to consider some of its more obvious physical characteristics. The first obvious feature of honey is its colour, which usually varies from almost water-white to nearly black.

The origin of this colour is not known. It may be due to carotenoids as these substances are frequently found in plants. It may possibly be due to certain polyphenolic substances such as tannins. Again these are universally present in plants and so would be transferred to honey from nectar. An early idea was that the colour was due to the caramelization of sugar. This now seems unlikely for when bees are confined to a room with access only to pure sugar syrup, the honey they make is always water-white. One would add, however, that when honey is heated, during industrial processing, for example, caramelization then contributes significantly to its colour.

Generally, honey colour is consistent with the plant source. So that water-white honey comes from oil-seed rape, pale white, having a tint of green, comes from willow-herb. Pale yellow honey is that from acacia, and intense golden yellow honey is from dandelion — a surprisingly rare honey in Britain. Lime honey has a pale greenish colour and honey with a rich port-wine colour is from heather.

As honey is normally graded on its appearance, colour is therefore of great importance in the honey business. In the past the honeys in greatest demand, particularly in Europe and North America, have been those of a pale colour. In general these also tend to be of a mild flavour. Colour also tends to be a reliable indicator of quality. Honeys from hot climates that may have been stored, for long periods, in dockside warehouses awaiting shipment, are generally dark. In addition the naturally acidic nature of honey tends to leach small amounts of iron from the metal containers in which it may be stored. Even those metal drums having a protective plastic internal coating are not immune to this problem. In the past Chinese exporters have tended to use inferior drums for honey storage so much so that Chinese honey is notorious for its high iron content. The presence of iron in honey tends to increase its overall pigmentation.

Additionally, the general conditions of hygiene under which honey is harvested has important consequences with regard to its colour. For example, if old honeycombs have been used in the beehive, particularly if previously they have held brood, then the honey will be considerably darker than if new combs had been employed. In Britain today the majority of beekeepers keep their honeycombs separate from those of the brood nest and so the honey is generally of a high standard. Needless to say, this does not apply to many overseas producers.

Some beekeepers, or honey packers, faced with the prospect of marketing a dark honey, may attempt to make it more acceptable by allowing it to crystallize, or 'set'. This results in a product that, because of its changed physical form will appear much lighter and so be more marketable.

Clarity

A further, if somewhat, dubious measure of honey quality is its clarity. Genuine honey is not normally perfectly clear. When held up to the light it should show a definite turbidity. On careful inspection there will be seen a vast array of tiny particles that include pollen grains, wax particles and other colloids, all being an integral part of the honey. As these substances enhance the nutritional value of honey they should not be removed by filtering. A brilliantly clear and transparent honey should therefore always be treated with caution.

It is relatively easy to check whether or not a honey has been finely sieved and filtered. A small amount of it is taken and dissolved in an equal volume of water. This is allowed to stand overnight in a tall glass. An unfiltered honey will deposit substantial sediment, whereas little will be evident if the honey has been filtered. If one has access to a simple microscope one can examine the sediment and study the pollen grains in more detail. The scientific name for this technique is melissopalynology. It is frequently employed by public analysts in their attempt to define the floral origin of a honey sample. Adulteration of a British honey with a foreign one may be detected by this method and the results obtained used in evidence of mislabelling.

Viscosity

Honey is a highly viscous substance. We all know how tedious it can be to take a spoonful without it dripping. However, with one honey this is not a problem — namely heather honey. If a jar of genuine heather honey is held up to the light one will see a mass of little air bubbles suspended in a gel which is normally port-wine in colour. The scientific name we give to this type of gel is 'thixotropic', a term familiar to most people in its application to non-drip paint. Thixotropic substances exist in a sort of semi-solid state that only becomes liquid on stirring. Heather honey is the only honey to have this property which is due to its high protein content.

Aroma

On opening a jar of honey we will be immediately aware of its unique aroma. This is due to the presence of a large variety of volatile organic substances that are mostly derived from nectar. Honey experts may frequently feel confident at being able to identify the source of a honey solely on account of its odour. This may, however, be misleading at times, particularly if it is a polyfloral honey in which one aroma may be masked by another.

Chemical Components

The chemical composition of honey is shown in Table 1.

Table 1

Average Composition of Honey

Component	*Average %*
Water	17
D-Fructose (levulose)	38
D-Glucose (dextrose)	32
Sucrose	1.3
Maltose	7.3
Higher sugars	1.5
Protein	0.3
Minerals	0.2
Vitamins, amino acids	1.0

Water

The average content of water in honey is somewhere between sixteen and twenty per cent; the exact content is important because at levels in excess of twenty per cent there is the likelihood of fermentation as honey is normally rich in osmophilic (sugar-liking) yeasts. Sometimes water is added to a dull honey to improve its clarity and give it a brilliant appearance. This may improve its selling potential but nevertheless is a form of adulteration and as such is illegal. Another reason why an individual might be tempted to do this is to make it easier to filter the honey. However, it must be stated, this practice is not widespread.

Sugars

Almost ninety-five per cent of the dry weight of honey consists of carbohydrates, or sugars. Honey, in fact, may be thought of as a concentrated solution of sugars in water. The principal sugars are glucose and fructose. Their ratio varies and is an important characteristic of an individual honey. In many multifloral honeys these two sugars are present in almost equal proportions, with perhaps a slight excess of fructose. On the other hand, many unifloral honeys contain more of one than the other. Rape honey, for example, contains more glucose than fructose and so granulates very quickly after harvesting. This is because glucose has a lower solubility in water than does fructose.

In contrast acacia honey has a greater proportion of fructose and so tends to remain in the liquid form almost indefinitely. Sucrose (that is ordinary table sugar) is also present in honey to the level of about one per cent. Some honeys, however, may have more, particularly some Australian honeys, and also where the beekeeper has overfed his bees with sugar. Overfeeding with sugar is again a form of adulteration and is relatively common in Britain. Although most beekeepers will vehemently protest their innocence, the following story illustrates their naivety.

In the late 1960's the Ministry of Agriculture made available 'denatured sugar' to beekeepers at a reduced cost. This was for feeding to bees and consisted of ordinary table sugar to which had been added a harmless green dye, so as to ensure it was not misused. When the beekeepers came to harvest their honey they were all amazed to discover it was blue-green in colour. This aroused considerable speculation and led to a protracted correspondence in the columns of the *Times* of February, 1971, until it was finally realised that it was a result of overfeeding with the cut-price sugar.

Mineral Content

The mineral content of honey varies from about 0.04 per cent in light coloured honey to 0.2 per cent in dark honey. The principal minerals are potassium, calcium, magnesium and silica. The exact mineral content will ultimately depend upon the type of soil in which the original nectar-bearing plant was located. In general, flower honeys have a lower mineral content than those from heaths and forests.

Honey is strongly acidic in nature and so should not be stored in metallic containers. Many honeys that are imported into Britain are transported in steel drums and the tendency is for the honey to slowly leach out iron from the container. Internal plastic layers are frequently used but they have limited usefulness, particularly as the drums are heated in order to liquify the contents. Furthermore, previous cleaning agents such as strong detergents may alter the protective layer sufficiently as to allow the acidic honey to attack the metallic surface beneath. Chinese honey, which is imported in substantial quantities into this country, is notorious for its high iron content.

Amino Acids

Honey contains a large number of different amino acids. These are, with the exception of proline, all derived from floral nectar. Thus, as each nectar has its own unique combination of amino acids, it is possible, using amino acid analysis, to determine the floral source of the nectar from which any particular honey is derived. This frequently may be used to indicate the likely geographical origin of a sample of honey.

Proteins

Most honey contains less than one half of a per cent of protein. Heather honey is exceptional in that it contains about one per cent. A small portion of the proteins in honey are enzymes. Although only small amounts are present only minute quantities are necessary for their biological activity. The major enzymes in honey are:

Invertase

This is the most abundant enzyme in honey and is derived from the hypophargyngeal gland of the bee. Its function is to break down sucrose into a mixture of glucose and fructose.

Diastase

This is probably derived from the floral nectar and its function is to break down starch into smaller sugars.

Glucose Oxidase

This is probably derived from the hypopharyngeal gland of the bee. This enzyme oxidises glucose, converting it into gluconic acid, with the production of hydrogen peroxide.

Catalase

Plants are rich in this enzyme, so it is likely that catalase in honey is derived from nectar. Its function is to break down hydrogen peroxide into water and oxygen.

Specific enzymes have, for a considerable time, been the basis of assessing honey quality. The reasoning behind this is that honey that has been adulterated, or overheated, will have a significantly reduced enzymatic activity.

Although the presence of enzymes in honey is a characteristic that sets it apart from other sweeteners, it nevertheless must be made clear that their presence can have no nutritional significance for man. It is well known that when enzymes are heated their activity is gradually lost, however, it would be unreasonable to argue that on account of this loss alone, that heated honey is somewhat less valuable to man than that which is unheated.

Vitamin Content

Most vitamins are present in honey at very low concentration and there is considerable variation depending upon the floral source. As the origin of the vitamins in honey is most likely to be the pollen, honey that has been filtered will have a low vitamin content. Some honeys have a high vitamin C content and these may contribute significantly to the daily requirements of this vitamin. However, in general, the vitamin levels in honey are so low as to have little nutritional significance.

Miscellaneous Constituents

More than 120 volatile substances have been identified in honey and they are thought to contribute to its aroma and flavour. Benzaldehyde and phenol have also been found in honey but they result from careless beekeeping procedures. These two substances are used by many beekeepers as bee repellants. The beekeeper uses a cloth soaked in one of them and places it over the honeycombs, so driving away all the bees, prior to him taking the harvest. If the beekeeper applies too much of the chemical it inevitably contaminates the honey.

Drugs used to treat bee diseases may also find their way into honey. Oxytetracycline, an antibiotic used to treat American Foul Brood Disease, has been found in some imported honeys. In Britain this disease is controlled by destroying infected colonies hence home-produced honey does not carry this risk.

Honey is a naturally acidic substance having a pH value between three and four. This acidity contributes towards its resistance toward the growth of micro-organisms. Much of this acidity is due to the presence of so-called 'plant acids' that include maleic acid, citric acid, oxalic acid, which are all derived from the nectar. The main acid however is gluconic acid which is produced from glucose by the action of the enzyme glucose oxidase.

This survey illustrates the variety of chemical compounds present in honey and although it is not intended to be an exhaustive survey, it nevertheless illustrates the complex composition of honey.

CHAPTER 5

Honey as a Commodity

In Britain we tend to have the misconception that life was much simpler in the past than it is today. Honey, in particular, tends to be associated with a rather nostalgic feeling for the 'good old days'. At the very mention of bees and honey, we immediately picture the sun beaming on a little thatched cottage, surrounded by pretty flowers, and a beehive in the background. I suppose we all yearn for some previous pre-industrial society, that has been conjured up in our imaginations largely from reading romantic literature. So, we tend to think of the sleepy English village, with its picturesque spire, and cricket match on the green. Such an image has been immortalized in the poem of Rupert Brooke that includes the famous lines:

> Oh! yet
> Stands the Church clock at ten to three?
> And is there honey still for tea?'

In this chapter we will look at how honey is presented to the public as a food commodity, how it is marketed, packaged and sold. But before we do this it is useful to appreciate some of the laws relating to its sale to the public.

Honey for Sale

The regulations that concern the sale of honey are probably the least restrictive of any that control the sale of food to the public. One reason for this is that honey is the least likely food to cause illness, or transmit disease to man. The recorded incidence of illness in man as a direct result of consuming honey is very small indeed. This is much more remarkable when one considers the fact that the honey most people eat has been produced in odd back-corners of fields and forests throughout the world.

And that there is absolutely no check on how it is harvested, collected or processed. The thousands of tons of honey imported each year into Britain has been collected under circumstances we know very little about.

Even in this country there is little, or no, supervision, or even regulations controlling honey production. There is not even a register of beekeepers. Anyone can set himself up as a beekeeper and sell whatever he thinks is honey to the public.

The few regulations that do exist are mainly concerned with labelling. Thus all honey on sale to the public must be labelled with the name and address of the producer, or packer. The one exception to this is when an individual beekeeper sells honey directly from his home. However, I believe that very few beekeepers who are proud of their produce would miss an opportunity of attaching their name to it. A label, however, must also have an accurate description of the contents of the jar. It must give the accurate weight and, if appropriate, the floral source of the honey.

Unfortunately there are few commercial fields of activity where some sharp practice does not exist. Honey is not one of them. Thus we find, particularly in some tourist areas, widespread misrepresentation. This might involve passing off a cheap imported honey for a locally produced one. The label may have been deliberately designed to mislead. It could feature a local landmark, or area, but in some obscure part of the label, (usually printed in small type) will be the words: 'produce of more than one country'.

Another type of fradulent mislabelling is where there might be a delightful picture of an orchard with the implication that the honey is from apple blossom, but in reality the jar contains some cheap imported honey. This sort of malpractice, although illegal, has gone on widely in the past.

Some commercial companies have tended to take advantage of the myth and mystery that surrounds honey in the imagination of the general public. Others play upon the widespread ignorance that exists. Thus we frequently find labels proclaiming such things as: 'Pure Organic Honey', or, 'Wild Flower Honey' and 'From bees fed only honey' and so on. All these statements are completely meaningless.

Mr Harold Inglesent, one time adviser to the World Health Organisation on nutritional matters, spent many years attempting to clean up the honey business. This lively octogenarian once told me how he would go around some of the most exclusive shops in the country and buy sample jars of honey. These he would take to his private laboratory and subject them to careful analysis. Frequently he would find that the description on the label did not match what was in the jar. Although he would return to the shop and complain, and no doubt cause considerable annoyance, he found it virtually impossible to change the lax attitudes that existed.

Liquid Honey

Firstly, the most popular form of honey is the runny, or liquid, variety. Unfortunately this preference by the general public for this type of honey has presented, and still does present, a major headache for the honey packers. The reason for this is that it is relatively difficult to keep liquid honey in this form for any length of time. The large commercial packing companies need to predict future sales with some accuracy, otherwise the liquid honey on the retailer's shelf will soon turn into unpleasant crystalline material that will render it unsaleable.

For a honey to have a reasonable shelf-life it needs to have been heated so that all 'seed' crystals have been dissolved. If this is not done the honey will slowly deposit unsightly crystals of glucose hydrate, with the consequence that the retailer will experience difficulty in selling it. By heating honey the little 'seed' crystals are forced to dissolve as the temperature rises. However, it is not possible to remove all 'seed' material, as small particles of dust, wax and pollen grains may also act as nuclei for the growth of glucose crystals. Honey manufacturers therefore go further and try to remove all these particles by employing pressure filtration devices. To accomplish this filtration in the least possible time and so save money, the honey is further heated to enable to to flow more easily through the filters. As we will discuss in detail in a later chapter, heating honey considerably reduces its nutritional value. On the other hand, home-produced honey has not been subjected to this type of processing and is consequently of much greater nutritional value. In addition, removing the pollen also detracts value from the honey, which as a natural product should be rich in pollen. Indeed, pollen should be regarded as an integral component of honey and should not be removed in this way. But as mentioned above, this dilemma is presented to the honey manufacturers as a consequence of the public's demand for liquid honey.

A further irrational demand by the public is for honey to be not only runny but for it to be sparklingly clear. Clarity is seen to be a sign of goodness in the product. This, however, is just the reverse of what it should be. Honey, because it contains pollen grains, particles of wax and so on, should not be of high clarity. As this misconception is widespread in the general public some individuals have been tempted to add water to their honey, both in an attempt to produce a honey of high clarity, and to assist in the filtration of it. Although such activity is illegal it would be exceedingly difficult to prove and hence prosecutions have been extremely rare.

Honey for use in medicine should not have been heated in any way at all. If it has been filtered it should have only been through a coarse filter, such as cheese cloth, that would leave its full complement of pollen. Honey that has been heated and pressure filtered is valueless from a medical and nutritional point of view. A jar of syrup, at around a third of the price, would probably be of equivalent value.

Set, or Granulated, Honey

When a scientist looks at honey he sees it as a supersaturated solution of glucose in water. The term 'supersaturated' simply means a solution in which more of the solute (in this case the glucose) has been dissolved than would normally do so at that particular temperature. Thus a supersaturated solution is relatively unstable and in time the excess solute, glucose in the case of honey, will come out of solution. Thus we find that liquid honey deposits crystals of glucose quite readily. Once crystals have begun to be deposited, crystallization will continue until the honey is completely crystallized, or granulated as it is sometimes called. If this process is uncontrolled, as it would be if, for example, it took place during the time the particular jar of honey stood on the retailer's shelf, then the net result would lack aesthetic appeal. Furthermore, as the crystals would tend to be rather large and hard it would be unpleasant to eat. In order to circumvent these difficulties the honey packers have increasingly tried to persuade the public to buy 'set' honey, which is a form of granulated honey in which the crystallization has occurred under controlled conditions.

To accomplish successfully the large-scale controlled crystallization of honey is not only a highly skilled operation, but also one that is largely unpredictable. It is absolutely crucial to get the right texture of crystals, and this is more of an art than a science. If the crystals are too large the granulated honey becomes rock hard, and the product in the trade would be referred to as a 'spoon-bender'. To be successful the crystallization must be controlled in such a way that the crystals formed are of a small uniform size. The resulting product is sometimes referred to as a 'creamed' honey. The process requires careful 'seeding', in which an already crystalline honey is ground up into tiny crystals and pumped into the bulk of the honey maintained at an appropriate temperature in a large tank. Mixing is then carefully carried out and the honey bottled directly. The jars of honey are then stored at an ambient temperature to allow the process to go to completion.

The introduction of 'creamed' honey has been a successful marketing ploy by the manufacturers, however problems still remain. In particular, as the honey market is very unpredictable, a jar of honey might, for instance, sit on a retailer's shelf for several weeks, and show signs of ageing. The usual indication of this is the so-called 'frosting' effect which is sometimes apparent in jars of honey. The problem of frosting arises directly from allowing the honey to granulate within the jar. As the honey sets from the centre and moves outwards there is an overall shrinkage. This tends to leave a tiny air gap at the interface of the inner surface of the jar and the surface of the honey. In time white crystals of glucose will slowly begin to appear and grow into shapes like frost crystals, hence its name. From a nutritional point of view, honey showing signs of frosting is equivalent to a freshly bottled one, but the customer does not see it like that, indeed he is usually put off by its appearance thinking that in some way the honey has 'gone off'.

Comb Honey

If honey is to be used in medicine then it is preferable to purchase it in comb form. Comb honey is usually available in three forms:

1. Section honey;
2. Cut-comb honey; and
3. Chunk-comb honey.

Comb honey in sections is without doubt the most attractive and medically useful form of honey. But producing section honey in its familiar wooden section boxes is not easy. It not only requires considerable skill on the part of the beekeeper but it is only best accomplished using a particular strain of bee.

In the past our own native strain of bee was best for producing section honey, but as today this bee is almost extinct, the production of section honey has consequently declined. This decline, which began earlier this century, has made it virtually impossible to obtain home-produced section honey. In general, the sections available in our shops today are produced in New Zealand.

The production problems arise because the beekeeper, in order to produce section honey, has to force his bees to occupy the tiny wooden boxes, which are normally held in racks above the main body of the hive. Bees are reluctant to do this and for the beekeeper to get any degree of success he must keep his bees in overcrowded conditions. This tends to encourage swarming, which gives the beekeeper further problems.

In addition to these problems the beekeeper must ensure that his bees only collect nectar from certain plants. As section honey would be unsaleable if it turned from the liquid form to the granulated type, he must make sure that his bees collect nectar from flowers that produce a honey that does not granulate. Because in Britain today we grow enormous quantities of oil-seed rape, which produces a honey that granulates very quickly, the beekeeper producing section honey has great difficulty in ensuring that none of this is collected by his bees.

In recent years there has appeared on the market a new variety of comb honey, known as 'cut-comb' honey. This is an excellent innovation and is a good way of purchasing unprocessed honey. The beekeeper produces this variety of honey by using entirely conventional honeycombs within his hive, except that they are fitted with very thin wax foundation and without wire struts. Once the entire honeycomb has been filled with honey and 'capped' the beekeeper lifts it out of the hive and then using a special metal cutter dissects it up into neat portions which he packs into small flat plastic containers ready for direct sale.

A third variety of comb honey is that available in jars with liquid honey normally referred to as 'chunk-comb' honey. Essentially this is clear honey, usually acacia honey, in which there is a piece of comb honey inserted. It is hardly ever produced by beekeepers and is more frequently offered for sale by commercial honey packers. Presumably they have adopted this type of marketing in the belief that the customer on seeing a piece of honeycomb within the jar will have confidence that the honey actually is genuine.

Honey Cappings

A final form of honey available is known as 'cappings'. These may be purchased from both beekeepers or from health food shops. In essence they are the wax cappings taken off the honeycomb prior to the extraction of the honey. There is usually plenty of honey mixed with them so that they may be eaten directly or used in much the same way as honey.

The beeswax, if eaten, is perfectly harmless and as the cappings are normally rich in pollen, the mixture is highly nutritious. Cappings are frequently recommended to be used in the treatment of hayfever and we will deal with this in detail in a later chapter.

CHAPTER 6

Varieties of Honey

Honeybees collect nectar from many thousands of different species of plant. Each nectar has its own individual characteristics that produce a honey unique in both aroma and flavour. Honey is known as 'monofloral' if it is produced exclusively from flowers of one species. Strictly speaking such a honey would be rare and normally, for practical purposes a monofloral honey is understood to be one in which the nectar of one particular plant predominates. An example is oil-seed rape honey, which almost always contains small amounts of nectar from other plants, that are not normally sufficient to influence its specific fragrance, flavour, or overall composition. On the other hand, honey produced from several floral sources is termed 'polyfloral'. This is distinct from blended honey, which is honey from different sources, both botanical and geographical, that have been mixed together by a honey packer. This is normally carried out by some of the large commercial concerns with the purpose of improving the flavour and appearance of inferior honeys. Thus to improve a dark honey, it would be blended with a pure white one, so converting it into a more marketable paler honey. In another instance the flavour of oil-seed rape honey might be improved by adding to it a darker and more strongly flavoured honey. Blending may also be carried out in order to alter the water content of a honey and so improve its shelf-life. To do this a honey with a low water content would be mixed with one having a high content of water. Blending honey is an extremely complex business that always carries the risk that a superior honey might be completely spoiled if the blending is inexpertly performed.

Let us now look in detail at the main types of honey produced in Britain. In general, British honeys are polyfloral, but there are a small number of unifloral varieties produced, these include the following.

Rape Honey

A little over ten years ago rape honey was virtually unknown in this country. In 1975 there were only about 10,000 acres of oil-seed rape grown in Britain, whereas in 1985 this acreage has increased to over 750,000. This remarkable increase has largely been brought about by the introduction of substantial subsidies offered to farmers to grow this crop. The result is that today it is very difficult to drive along our motorways during the summer without seeing the, now familiar, blaze of yellow somewhere in the distance. Unfortunately, British beekeepers have been slow to take advantage of this valuable source of nectar. If it were to be fully exploited by beekeepers, Britain could become self-sufficient in honey production.

The production of rape honey does however present a number of problems for beekeepers. It is a honey that has a very high glucose content and so tends to crystallize, or granulate, very quickly after harvesting. If it is not bottled immediately after taking off the hive it tends to granulate in the comb and so become ruined. Many beekeepers, in their attempt to avoid this mishap, harvest rape honey before it has been capped by the bees. This is then immature, or 'unripe', honey, which has such a high water content that it tends to quickly ferment.

As all rape honey granulates so quickly, most that is on sale in our shops will invariably be the 'set' variety. In appearance it will be very pale white with an insipid flavour that, because of its high content of glucose, is unpleasantly sweet for most palates.

In 1982, the University of Salford carried out a national survey of honey in collaboration with the British Beekeepers' Association. In this survey, in which I participated, we came across many samples of rape honey that were actively fermenting. We had originally supplied the beekeepers with small airtight plastic containers for them to place their samples of honey, but we found in our laboratory that these containers soon presented a 'blown' appearance, characteristic of fermenting honey.

Fortunately during the last couple of years farmers have been trying out new varieties of oil-seed rape that have been found to yield a honey that does not granulate so quickly. When more of this crop is cultivated the problem of rape honey being prematurely removed from the hive will largely be over.

Heather Honey

This is a highly flavoured honey that is the pride of Scotland. It is usually a beautiful rich port-wine colour that has a bitter-sweet taste appealing to the discerning palate. Demand for genuine heather honey is high and so normally is its price.

As has been discussed in a previous chapter heather honey is renowned for its thixotropic character, so that under normal conditions it is a solid gel and only becomes liquid on stirring. This characteristic makes it tedious for the beekeeper to extract from the comb and is why many beekeepers prefer to sell heather honey in the comb.

Those beekeepers who do extract heather honey do so by wrapping the honeycombs in cheese cloth and squeezing out the honey in a honey press. This is both time-consuming and messy. Although demanding considerable patience, the product, when it is obtained, is certainly worth it, as heather honey is really delicious.

Pressed honey, as it contains a full complement of pollen, is excellent from a nutritional point of view. Usually, during the pressing operation, a considerable amount of air bubbles become incorporated so giving the honey a characteristic and pleasing appearance. When purchasing this type of honey one should always ensure it has this unique feature. In the past many blended honeys have been passed off as 'heather' honey, so on purchasing heather honey one should ensure that it:

1. is thixotropic;
2. contains suspended air bubbles; and
3. has not granulated.

These remarks, however, should be qualified in that heather honey from the moors and heathlands of Southern England may occasionally granulate.

Willow Herb Honey

This is one of the finest and most delicious honeys produced in Britain. It has a most delicate aroma and flavour, and in appearance is pale with a slight greenish tinge.

The willow-herb plant, is also known as rosebay, or fireweed. To many people it is considered a weed as it tends to grow profusely on wasteland. After the last war its characteristic tall, elegant, rose-red flowers were to be seen over many of the bomb sites in our major cities. Now the same sentinels guard our industrial wastelands. As it is an excellent honey-producing plant these inner city areas are now a source of bumper crops of honey for the urban beekeeper.

In contrast to rape honey, willow herb honey is very slow to granulate and jars purchased in September are usually still liquid the following summer. However, as it is so delicious, it is much more likely for it to have been consumed long before then.

Clover Honey

At one time this was the major variety of honey produced in Britain. In recent years, however, its production has declined due to the gradual loss of the old permanent pastures.

In appearance clover honey is pale straw in colour. It has a delightful aroma. But it tends to granulate quickly and the crystals formed are usually small and hard. Set clover honey therefore tends to be of a rigid texture and so is rather unpleasant.

Lime Honey

This is one of the world's finest and most sought after honeys. It is highly valued both for its magnificent flavour and its fragrance. Lime honey usually has a greenish-yellow colour and when freshly extracted is of high clarity.

In Britain it is frequently produced by the many urban beekeepers who are able to place their hives near to the many lime trees that grow in our public parks. Lime trees secrete nectar profusely which is collected by bees providing atmospheric conditions of temperature and humidity are suitable. If, on a warm day in July, one stands beneath a lime tree, once can hear the combined hum of the myriads of bees busily engaged in collecting the lime nectar. In such circumstances it is easy to realize how the lime tree became known as the 'queen' of honey plants.

Raspberry Honey

The main area in Britain producing raspberry honey is Eastern Scotland around Dundee. This variety of honey has a fine delicate flavour and aroma. In appearance it is pale white. Unfortunately it tends to granulate quickly, forming very small crystals of glucose hydrate.

Other Varieties

The above are the major monofloral honeys produced in Britain. Some of the other varieties which are not so common are listed and described in Table 2.

Table 2

Some Other British Unifloral Honeys

Plant	***Characteristics of the Honey***
Blackberry/Bramble	Although wild blackberry is ubiquitous in this country, pure blackberry honey is extremely rare. When it is found it is dark amber in colour and granulates quickly.
Hawthorn	Hawthorn honey is very rich in flavour, but it is only rarely obtained as a unique monofloral honey. It is usually deep amber in colour.
Broad Bean	Beekeepers who keep their hives near to fields where this crop is grown are able to obtain this honey as a monofloral variety. Its characteristics however are rather variable. A lot seems to depend upon the local soil. Sometimes it is very dark, with a strong flavour whereas in other seasons it is very light with a delicate flavour. Possibly it is occasionally collected along with honeydew.
Sycamore	This honey is light amber in colour with a greenish tinge. Usually one finds that its flavour tends to mature over several months, so it is best not to consume it too early. It is rarely pure sycamore honey and is most likely to be mixed with other spring flowers.
Sainfoin	At one time sainfoin was extensively grown in this country for fodder, but today very little is cultivated. The honey when it is obtained has a bright golden colour. It has an exceedingly pleasant aroma with a delightful flavour.
Dandelion	Surprisingly, dandelion honey is quite rare in Britain. When it is obtained its colour varies from bright golden yellow to amber. It has an excellent flavour but its aroma is rather strong.

Dandelion honey granulates soon after it is extracted to form large coarse crystals that render it rather unattractive.

Sea Lavender Sea lavender honey is only produced along the salt marshes of the East Coast. It has an exceptional flavour and in colour is light to medium amber.

World Production of Honey

The annual world production of honey is about a million tons. More than half of this is produced by the three largest beekeeping countries, namely, the United States, the USSR and China. Other large producers are Australia, Argentina, Mexico and Canada. Britain, and most other European countries, are net importers of honey. Some of the characteristics of honey imported into Britain from these countries is summarized below.

Australian Honey

Australia is one of the main sources of honey imported into Britain. The standards of hygiene under which Australian honey is produced are excellent. Strict quality control measures are enforced and only honey satisfying the rigorous standards of the Australian Honey Board is permitted to be exported.

Chinese Honey

China is now a major producer and exporter of honey. According to the latest Overseas Trade Statistics almost one-fifth of honey imported into Britain is of Chinese origin. Many varieties are produced, including buckwheat, lime and acacia. Unfortunately the standards maintained for its packaging and export have left much to be desired. Many of the drums used for transport have been found to be rather battered and rusting. Consequently Chinese honey has been notorious for its high iron content.

Mexican Honey

Since the last war Mexico has become one of the leading honey-producing nations. However, standards of production in some areas are still primitive, consequently some Mexican honeys are of poor quality.

Russian Honey

Russia produces a great variety of honey, much of it of a very high quality. Unfortunately only a little is imported into Britain. The standards of production are good and the conditions employed in the export of Russian honey are excellent.

American Honey

Only a small amount of American honey is imported into Britain. The notable feature about American honey is that it is always highly sieved and filtered so consequently it is usually completely free of pollen. From a nutritional point of view this is undesirable and it is difficult to understand why the manufacturers go to such lengths. Even honey sold for cooking has had the pollen removed.

Hungarian Honey

Hungary is notable for its production and export of acacia honey. The quality and purity of this honey is excellent. As it will remain liquid almost indefinitely, in most cases it will not have been heated during processing and bottling. This honey is therefore preferable to other commercial varieties.

Table 3

Characteristics of some Imported Honeys

Plant	*Geographical Origin*	*Features*
Acacia	Hungary, Romania, Yugoslavia	Acacia honey is a pale yellow colour, having a very mild flavour. As it is high in fructose it will remain liquid almost indefinitely. Because of this it is frequently used as the liquid honey in the variety of honey known as chunk-comb honey.
Eucalyptus	Australia	Eucalyptus honey is light amber in colour with a strong flavour. It is renowned for its medical properties and in particular has been widely used to treat chest complaints.

Clover	New Zealand, Canada	When pure, imported clover honey is very similar to that produced in Britain.
Rosemary	Spain	Rosemary honey is both delicious and delicate in flavour.
Banksia	Australia	Banksia honey is notable for its oversweet taste which is on account of its high sucrose content.
Alfalfa	USA	Alfalfa honey is light amber in colour, and has a mild flavour and pleasant aroma. As it is slow to granulate it is frequently sold as comb honey. Because of its mild flavour, honey packers tend to blend it with darker more strongly flavoured honeys.
Basswood	USA	Basswood honey has a water-white appearance and distinctive minty flavour. It is usually slow to granulate, so makes excellent comb honey.
Buckwheat	China, USA	Buckwheat honey is jet-black in appearance and when unprocessed contains an abundance of bright yellow pollen. It has a very strong flavour, so much so, that many honey packers blend it with milder honeys before putting it on the market. It normally has a high iron content and so is frequently recommended for patients suffering with anaemia. Traditionally it has been used to treat bronchial disorders.
Goldenrod	USA	Goldenrod honey has a rich, deep yellow colour. It is a thick, heavy honey with a strong flavour. It has the disadvantage that it granulates quickly.

Sage	USA	Sage honey is pure white in colour with a delicate aroma. It is slow to granulate.
Citrus	Spain, Israel, Malta, USA	Most citrus honeys are marketed as 'orange blossom honey' even if they have originated from lime, lemon, or grapefruit. Generally they have a pale colour with a mild but distinctive flavour.
Yellow Box	Australia	Yellow Box honey has a pale yellow appearance with a very mild flavour. As it has a high fructose content it granulates very slowly.
Blue Gum	Australia	Blue Gum honey is very dark in appearance with both a pleasant flavour and bouquet.
Leatherwood	Tasmania	Leatherwood honey is famous for its delightful flavour. It is usually light amber in colour and tends to granulate very slowly.
Thyme	Greece	Wild thyme honey, or Hymettus honey, has been known since antiquity as 'food of the gods'. It usually has a reddish colour and strong distinctive flavour.

Honeydew

There is considerable confusion amongst the general public as to what exactly honeydew is. Many people buy it in the belief that it is another variety of honey. It should at the outset be stated that honeydew is *not* a form of honey. Honey can only be considered to be such if it is from plant nectar. Honeydew is simply not derived from plant nectar and so is *not* honey. Not only is there confusion in the public but there is also ignorance in the people who draft out our legislation, for the British laws relating to honey, namely *The Honey Regulations* (1976), make the mistake of calling honeydew honey. The actual wording states that 'honeydew . . . means honey' and then goes on to describe honey as: 'a fluid viscous, or crystallized food which is produced by honeybees from nectar of blossoms or from secretions of, or *found on* living parts of plants, other than blossoms . . .'. Both of these descriptions are inaccurate. Honeydew is honeydew and not honey. This is not simply being pedantic, but is of some importance, as these laws define what is considered to be human food. Many people have maintained the view that as honeydew is derived from an insect excrement it is not suitable as a human food and I entirely agree with them. On the other hand, those individuals who advocate its use as a part of our diet prefer to see honeydew in euphemistic terms as being 'exuded by plant-sucking insects'. Whereas, in fact, honeydew is *excreted* by plant-sucking insects. These insects are usually aphids that live on plants by damaging their tissue and sucking the sap. Their excrement contains unwanted sugars which are collected by bees.

In my view honeydew should not be classed as honey, nor should it be considered as a wholesome food. For one reason, as it is a very sticky substance, that lies about on the leaves of trees for some considerable time before it is collected by bees, it will inevitably pick up environmental pollutants. In cities, for example, this will be lead from car exhausts, and industrial pollutants (some of them carcinogenic). These will be absorbed by this sticky material. Eventually these will contaminate the honeydew that is collected by the beekeeper. Indeed chemical analysis of honeydew has demonstrated that it has a high inorganic content.

In comparison, the collection of nectar is from the interior part of the plant, that it is not exposed to the environment for any length of time, and the honey produced is comparatively free of these environmental pollutants.

A further unpleasant aspect of honeydew is that it is usually contaminated with the spores and mycelium of a black sooty mould that grows on foliage that is covered in this aphid excrement. So that, when it is collected by bees they also collect this mould, which becomes incorporated into the 'honey' of the hive.

CHAPTER 7

Honey Production Past and Present

The methods of honey production first adopted by the ancient Egyptians and then developed by the Greeks remained virtually unchanged until a century, or so, ago. In a previous chapter we have seen how the ancient Egyptians harvested their honey by filtering it through linen cloth and then storing it in earthenware vessels. For centuries this procedure remained unchanged, and so we must presume that honey produced in this way is that which throughout antiquity has been associated with medical value. We cannot equate the mass-produced honey, that is sold in retail outlets today, with that produced in antiquity. How do the production methods differ?

There are two important differences: firstly, the honey produced in ancient times was virtually unheated; and secondly, it was either eaten on the comb, or squeezed through coarse cloth. This type of honey would therefore retain a full complement of pollen.

As we will see in a subsequent chapter, mass-produced honey is subjected to considerable heating. Furthermore, beekeeping techniques employed today are such that all honey harvested has a low pollen count. In the past this would not have been the case. Centrifugal extractors are used today even by the smallest beekeeper when removing honey from the honeycombs. This technique ensures that large amounts of pollen remain behind in the comb and so are not incorporated into the honey. In addition many honey packers use filters that remove any trace of pollen that may remain in the honey.

Let us examine in detail the production methods employed today and compare them with those used in the past.

For many centuries the monasteries were centres of beekeeping, as they were also of medicine. Indeed even before the Christian era, beekeeping is believed to have been a major occupation of the monastic Essenes.

Hives, or 'skeps' as they were known, were made from straw, or wickerwork, and bound together with bramble. Inside one of these the colony of bees would be protected from the elements. The bees would build combs that would be supported by the upper surface and walls so that it was impossible to remove the honey without disturbing them. In order to harvest the honey it was necessary to kill the bees. This would be carried out in the autumn when the beekeeper would have to decide which hives should be kept and which destroyed. A general rule was to take all the hives that were full of honey. Of the lighter ones only those three years old and older were taken. A hole would be dug in the ground and, in the evening, sulphur burned in it. The skep was placed over the pit and the bees poisoned by the fumes. When dead they were easily shaken from the combs and the honey drained into a large earthenware container. The honey was allowed to settle in the container and any wax debris that floated to the surface was removed. This honey was called 'virgin honey'. The remaining honeycombs were pressed to yield what was called 'common honey'. This contained, in addition to the pure honey, a great deal more pollen. The combs that remained after pressing were soaked in water and made into mead.

Many beekeepers were unhappy having to kill their bees and many attempts were tried to devise an alternative system of collecting the honey. One such method which some of our older beekeepers can still recall is 'driving' the bees. The skep containing the honey and colony would be inverted and an empty skep placed above it. The lower skep would be banged and smoked so as to force the bees up into the top one. Competitions of bee driving were a regular feature of many horticultural and agricultural shows until quite recently. Hence . . .

How doth the little busy Bee,
Increase her little power,
And gather favour every day,
And almost every hour!

How pleased she hears within her cell
That Apiculture thrives!
That honeycomb is selling well,
And Bees are having 'drives'.!

Punch 14 August 1880

By the early eighteenth century progressive beekeepers had devised more efficient methods. Thorley introduced simply box hives made of inch-thick deal in about 1730. These boxes were about ten inches deep and fourteen inches square. Bars were added across the top so that the bees could attach their combs. Windows were sometimes incorporated and even brass handles attached! Four such hives would be incorporated into a small beehouse that would protect them from the weather. To complete the picture red, white, blue, or yellow shapes in the form of half-moons, or squares, were painted on the outside so as to distinguish one colony from another. No doubt these were delightful decorative features in one's garden but from a beekeeper's point of view were rarely successful.

Around 1806 the Ukranian Peter Prokopovich developed what must be the first movable-frame hive. The bars had grooves in them so as to permit the bees passage from one chamber to another. However, the bees still glued the frames to the hive walls with propolis and made them virtually impossible to remove.

This situation remained until 1851 when the Rev Lorenzo Langstroth discovered and patented the idea of 'bee space'. By observing bees through glass hives Langstroth had noticed that bees would always leave a three-eighths of an inch space around the combs. He therefore designed a movable frame that provided for this space on all sides and discovered that the bees would rarely glue it to the hive walls. This was the first moveable frame which, soon after its introduction, revolutionized bee-keeping the world over.

The next significant invention also came from America. It was the centrifugal extractor and was first demonstrated in this country at the Crystal Palace Exhibition of 1874. It was called the 'Slinger', and it too soon became adopted by many beekeepers who realised that the extracted combs could be reused.

Although considerably speeding up the extraction process, the introduction of the mechanical extractor may be looked upon as a retrograde step in the history of honey production. By using it beekeepers tended to continually reuse their honeycombs, some after having been stored in far from hygienic conditions. Even today beekeepers, in their attempt to save money, tend to use unsuitable combs. Furthermore, as the wax moth is a problem when storing combs, beekeepers tend to treat the combs with the insecticide p-dichlorobenzene, which acts as a wax moth repellant. Inevitably this chemical gets absorbed by the wax of the combs and eventually contaminates the honey. As this chemical is toxic to man, its presence in honey can only do harm.

Thus the centrifugal extraction of honey leads to a different type of honey from that prepared in ancient times. It would have a low pollen count and, even if it had been obtained under the most scrupulous conditions, would be inferior from a medical point of view.

But by far the most important change has been the importing of vast quantities of foreign honey into this country. Although small amounts of foreign honey have always been imported into Britain, towards the end of the last century North American became a major producer of honey and began to export large quantities into Europe. Although initially the honey-bee was absent on the North American continent, after first being introduced by the early English settlers in about 1620 it soon spread over a vast area, so much so, that the native Indians referred to honey bees as 'white man's flies'. The vast areas of trees, shrubs and flowers all producing nectar in abundance allowed the honeybees to flourish. Honey soon began to be produced in enormous quantities and huge numbers of workers became engaged in this industry. By 1880 it was estimated that there were over a million hives throughout the country.

The journal *Nature* commented: 'We are led to understand how much this branch of industry is advancing in America, where honey is now being manufactured on almost as large a scale as corn' 9 September, 1880. And *Punch*, in an article headed 'Our little busy bees and their very busy American cousins' wrote: 'There has lately been a vehement protest of the British beekeepers against the influx of American honey. All flying insects in the States we know are called "Bugs". Naturally enough, indignant English Apiarians called the Yankee bees — Humbugs.' (22nd February 1879) The same pattern was to be repeated in Australia, New Zealand and, more lately, Mexico. Large amounts of honey began to be imported and with this there began a gradual decline in beekeeping activities in this country. Only during World War II was there an upsurge in interest, but since then home production of honey has steadily dwindled. Today more than ninety per cent of all honey consumed in Britain is imported.

To appreciate the significance of this we need to understand the vital difference between home-produced and imported honey. Although both are produced in similar ways there exists an important difference. The actual beehives vary only slightly. Overseas they are rather larger, but they all use moveable frames, and the honey is extracted, as in Britain, using centrifugal extractors. However, in isolated areas abroad the honey is stored in large containers to await collection for delivery to regional centres.

In Australia, and some other countries, export honey is prepared only in registered premises, which must meet certain minimum standards with regards to general hygiene. In some countries the standards are far better than those many British beekeepers employ. But the problem arises at the next stage. The honey is packed into forty-four-gallon steel drums and exported by sea. By the time it reaches this country and gets delivered to the honey packer much of it has granulated within the drum. To get it out it must be heated so as to render it liquid. To do this the lids are ripped off and the drum inverted in a large heated oven, where the honey, as it melts, is allowed to drain away.

The liquefied honey is fed into enormous settling tanks where blending with other honeys takes place. The honey is then pumped through filters and finally bottled. All this time the honey is maintained at a relatively high temperature.

In contrast to this, home-produced honey is bottled directly after it is extracted and may be with the consumer the day after it was taken from the hive. This is the crucial difference between home-produced honey and that which is imported. Only the former can be considered suitable for use in medicine.

CHAPTER 8

Honey for Use as a Medicine

The majority of people in Britain today see honey to be a rather pleasant item of food. This, however, is a somewhat recent view, for throughout history honey has been valued as an important therapeutic agent. As medicine is now dominated by the marketing devices of the drug companies, it is very convenient to dismiss as a 'myth' the medical value of honey. Even many beekeepers have been led to accept this view, which is promulgated in the current beekeeping literature.

I maintain the simple view that if home-produced honey were to be available in place of that mass-produced, the health of the British people would be vastly improved. The tragedy is that Britain could easily be self-sufficient in honey production. Unfortunately, again, people have been hoodwinked into believing that this also is a myth.

Effect of Heat on Honey

As we have discussed in the preceding chapter, the distinction between mass-produced and home-produced honey is that the former is heated. Throughout history the heating of honey has been thoroughly condemned. In ancient Egypt and Assyria there were severe penalties for any beekeeper found heating his honey. Extant records clearly show that honey must be 'untouched by fire'. The physicians in ancient Greece and throughout Mediaeval times all held this same view. As it is very convenient when working with honey to heat it, for example it makes the pouring of it very much easier, had these early peoples therefore discovered some empirical information that convinced them of its detrimental effects? In my opinion this seems very likely. So if honey is to be used in medicine today it must not have been heated to a temperature greater than that found within the hive, that is between ninety-five and ninety-seven degrees Fahrenheit.

The Fiehe's Test

Today we have a very simple colorimetric test known as the Fiehe's test which may detect honey that has been heated above this temperature. Recently I purchased ten jars of mass-produced honey, from different countries and companies. On doing the Fiehe's test on these samples I found every one to give a strong positive reaction. However, on repeating the test on ten samples of home-produced honey, obtained from different beekeepers, I found that not one gave even the slightest indication of a positive reaction. This simple test convinced me that there did exist an important difference between mass-produced and home-produced honey.

Heating to delay Fermentation

We have seen in the previous chapter how honey packers heat their honey to assist blending and filtering. But in addition they heat it as a form of pasteurization. This is to delay any possible fermentation if yeasts are present. To accomplish this the honey is heated at about 160 degrees Fahrenheit for about an hour. This renders the yeast cells inactive and enables the honey packer to sell his product to the retailer with some confidence that it won't ferment while standing on the shelf in his shop.

All this amounts to a considerable amount of heating and is well known to the authorities who for some time have maintained nominal standards. These standards relate to the loss of certain natural enzymes within the honey, in particular the enzyme diastase. During heating the activity of this enzyme is known to decrease, and it is this loss of activity that is used to signify how much the honey has been heated. These regulations however are not strictly imposed and there have been very few prosecutions for infringements.

HMF

A more reliable indicator of how much a honey has been heated is the level of the chemical 5-hydroxymethyl-2-furfuraldehyde (HMF). HMF is formed when honey is heated as a breakdown product of fructose. Much ignorance surrounds HMF both amongst honey packers and beekeepers.

The regulations at present indicate that honey cannot be sold if its HMF content is greater than 80 p.p.m. (p.p.m. standing for, parts per million). EEC regulations specify a level of 40 p.p.m. and it is nothing short of scandalous that our authorities have permitted the higher level. Indeed to make matters worse I understand that there is pressure from some honey importers to have an even higher upper limit. This would allow them to import cheaper honeys and to be able to heat the honey further during processing.

The fact remains that there are some honeys on the market today with HMF levels well above the legal maximum. Not only does this indicate that they have been severely heated, but that they may be a danger to health. HMF is a very dangerous chemical that should not be present in our food. It should certainly not be present in honey and *is not present* in freshly isolated home-produced honey.

There is very little known about the toxicity of HMF. We do know that when bees are fed sugar solutions containing trace amounts of HMF they quickly die. As long ago as 1948 Drs T. B. Heaton and G. B. Robinson of the University of Oxford reported in the October issue of *Nature* that minute amounts of HMF would arrest the growth of rats. This work has been largely ignored except for several groups of Russian scientists who have been concerned about HMF in the environment. These workers have discovered that on feeding HMF to rats extensive liver damage resulted.

Mass-produced honey that contains high levels of HMF should not be sold in our shops. In particular, as it may interfere with growth, it should not be eaten by children. This type of honey has no role to play in natural medicine.

CHAPTER 9

Honey for Hayfever and Asthma

Hayfever

Hayfever, or as it is known medically, 'pollinosis', or 'seasonal allergic rhinitis' (rhinitis being the technical term for a runny nose), is characterized by sneezing, nasal discharge and inflammation of the nasal mucous membranes. In the past this complaint has been referred to as 'Hay asthma', 'pollen catarrh', or 'rose-cold'.

We do not know whether hayfever has always afflicted mankind, or whether it is a relatively new disease. The earliest description of it occurs in 1803 when W. Heberden wrote in his book *Commentaries on the History and Cure of Disease* that 'summer catarrh' would return 'in four out of five persons annually in the months of April, May, June and July and last a month with great violence'. The next description was by Dr J. Bostock, who had suffered from it for forty-seven years and wrote in 1819 'experience of many years has taught me not to expect a cure for this complaint'. He called it 'Catarrhus Aestivus' and described it as a 'periodical affection of the eyes and chest'. He also mentions that the popular term for the complaint was 'hayfever'.

The first suggestion that it was caused by pollen was made by Dr J. Elliotson in 1831. However, the first systematic study was not made until 1862 when Dr Phillip Phoebus of Giessen carried out an extensive survey. Its cause, however, was not firmly established until Charles H. Blackley, a Manchester physician, published his classic work *Experimental Researches on the Causes and Nature of Cattarrhus Aestivus* in 1873. Blackley, who was also a sufferer, carried out many of his experiments on himself. Using careful scientific tests he showed that pollen was the sole cause and that the severity of the disease was related to the amount present in the atmosphere.

Today we view hayfever as the classic allergic disease. Its occurrence is now known to be world-wide. In the United States almost fifteen per cent of the population suffer from ragweed hayfever alone. In some Australian cities over ten per cent of the citizens are affected, but in Britain only around five per cent of the population are known to be sufferers. There are few complications of hayfever and death has not been recorded, however suicide from the depression that may accompany it has been known. The main culprits in this country are the flowering grasses, however, once hayfever has set in, inhaled pollen from any source may evoke further attacks. The pollens from grasses, weeds and trees are relatively light and when dry are easily blown about in the wind to cover both cities and countryside. In the United Kingdom the hayfever season lasts between 20 May and the 15 July, varying slightly with temperature and weather, whereas in the United States the season is rather longer.

An attack is evoked when pollen, varying in size from 10 microns to 100 microns is inhaled and becomes trapped in the mucous membranes of the nasal tract. The membranes become inflamed and swell up, so blocking the nasal passages. Respiration becomes difficult and there is profuse lacrymation. With time the discharge from the eyes and nose becomes thicker and infections may set in. Normally an attack may last for a few hours, several days, or even longer.

If one reads the findings of many of the early Victorian investigators one finds repeated reference to the disease having racial and occupational predisposition. People of Anglo-Saxon descent were frequently found to be sufferers, particularly if they were amongst the educated middle classes. Thus English people residing in India and Africa were frequently affected, but never the native peoples. Furthermore, professional people were frequent sufferers whereas agricultural workers who were continuously exposed to pollen never seemed to contract it. This puzzled physicians of the day and the *British Medical Journal* of 23 June, 1883 commented: 'one of the *curious* facts about hayfever is that it is especially common in the "well-to-do", while haymakers and others who work in hayfields are exempt!' Today we know differently. It is almost certain that these observations do not reflect the true epidemiology of the disease as only the wealthy had the time and money to attend a physician on account of a disease that most of the working classes would have dismissed as trivial. *Punch* commented on what it saw to be a 'Fashionable Epidemic' as follows:

> There is a curious epidemic flying about we hardly know what it is but it attacks principally the highest and the middle classes.
>
> So very contagious is it and so certain in its effects, that, to our knowledge alone, no less than 5632 families principally residing at the West End have been ordered by their physicians to leave town immediately for a 'change of air'.
>
> (*Punch*, 1853 vol. 25 p. 79)

It was indeed a fashionable disease and recommended treatments included holidays by the seaside, long sea voyages and extended stays in expensive Swiss mountain resorts. How many of the working classes, who were apparently immune to this disease, could afford such treatments?

Today, it is now evident that as Western society has become more affluent, so the incidence of hayfever has increased. It now affects double the number of people it did fifty years ago. Also, immigrants to Britain, who have never experienced it before, have become sufferers. It is therefore a disease associated with modern society and a disease probably unknown to primitive man.

As with so many other allergic diseases, psychosomatic factors play a significant role. Over a century ago Dr J. N. Mackenzie showed that a patient could have an attack on being exposed to an artificial flower.

Emotional stress in particular is involved. Students facing examinations frequently develop hayfever. One consultant physician, a sufferer for over forty years, wrote: 'while preparing for my third MB examination at the age of 20, I developed hayfever . . .' (BMJ 14 July 1979). Another doctor first developed it at the age of ten during a moment of stress in a preparatory school cricket match, and another severe attack while he was on honeymoon (BMJ 11 August 1979).

These observations were nothing new. A writer to the *British Medical Journal* in July 1883 concluded about hayfever: 'I think neurosis seems to underline most cases and to constitute the essential cause or predisposition on which the disease depends . . .'

–Perennial Allergic Rhinitis and Allergic Asthma–

Perennial allergic rhinitis, which is similar to hayfever, may occur at any time in the year. It is caused by inhalation of dust, animal danders, fungi spores, and so on. Today, almost one person in four, has some form of allergic illness and allergic rhinitis accounts for a large proportion of them.

Many of the allergens are derived from natural organic sources. Household dust, for example, is contaminated with the common dust mite, which is a notorious allergen. When these substances come into contact with the respiratory tract an allergic reaction similar to that described for hayfever ensues.

Both forms of allergic rhinitis may develop into asthma, which in turn may progress to the very serious condition known as emphysema. Only recently have we realised the importance of environmental chemicals in the development of these diseases, which constitute a growing problem for our society. Allergic asthma is in particular on the increase in young children, and is now the most frequent chronic illness amongst children both in Europe and America.

Asthma, unlike hayfever, has been known since antiquity. Indeed the word 'asthma' itself comes from the Greek for 'breathlessness', which sums it up quite well. In this disease there is a narrowing of the bronchial airways that may lead to sudden attacks of breathlessness and wheezing. Such attacks may change in severity over short intervals. Attacks of asthma, therefore, are intermittent. They are evoked by a combination of factors just as with hayfever. Any emotional stress at the time an allergen comes into contact with the respiratory system will make an acute attack more likely.

To appreciate hayfever, allergic rhinitis and asthma one needs some understanding of the allergic reaction. Much progress has been made in this field during the last twenty years, so much so, that the academic understanding of its mechanism has far outstretched the means of treatment.

The Immune Response

All allergens, whether they are pollen particles that induce hayfever or dust granules that trigger off perennial allergic rhinitis or asthma, have in common specific antigenic components within its molecular structure. Normally this is protein in nature. It is this section of the allergen that reacts with the mucosal surface of the respiratory tract. Normally what happens when, for example, a foreign protein allergen comes into contact with the body is for substances known as 'antibodies' to be produced. These quickly render the intruder substance harmless. For some unknown reason the reaction may follow either one of two pathways. One is along an immediate pathway leading to the formation of the antibody immunoglobulin E (IgE). The other is a delayed response which produces a different type of antibody known as immunoglobulin G (IgG).

In an allergic reaction contact with the allergen produces large amounts of the type one antibody, namely IgE. Soon after exposure to an allergen raised levels of IgE begin to circulate in the blood. These react with specific cells known as 'mast cells'. On binding with these cells biochemicals are released into the blood that have intense physiological activity. One such biochemical is histamine. It is histamine that brings about the symptoms of allergic disease such as wheezing, itching, inflammation and so on.

Antihistamines

One way to combat the release of histamine is to counteract its effects by specific drugs known as 'antihistamines'.

Each year millions of pounds are spent by the National Health Service on antihistamine drugs. These drugs work by blocking receptors for histamine on cells and so halting the histamine response. But as other substances, besides histamine, are released by the mast cells, they fail to cope adequately in controlling the response. As with many drugs they attempt to suppress the symptoms but do not treat the cause of the disease. Furthermore, many antihistamines have a sedating and disorienting effect that makes, for example, driving a car during treatment rather hazardous. Professional performance might also be affected. One Cambridge surgeon wrote to the *British Medical Journal* in June 1951 describing how, when he was being treated with antihistamines for hayfever, he found great difficulty getting dressed after a morning in the operating theatre. He was so severely disoriented that it took him half an hour to tie his tie!

The *British Medical Journal* has reported that according to a survey they conducted between half and three-quarters of all cases of hayfever gradually develop into asthma if antihistamines are relied on. This statistic does question the usefulness of these drugs and warrants a search for an alternative solution.

Drug Treatment

Drug companies have not been slow in seeking and introducing drugs to treat these illnesses. The so-called 'wonder-drug' cortisone was found to be extremely effective in reducing allergic inflammation. This led to the development of a large number of new corticosteriod drugs. They could be administered in tablet form, injection or inhaled and were found to be effective in relieving bronchial spasm and inflammation in cases of allergic asthma. These drugs have also been used to treat hayfever. Side effects were, however, quickly recognized. These included: hypertension; weight gain; susceptibility to fungal infections; and cataract formation. In children growth retardation was found to occur. Although attempts were made to limit these disadvantages they could not altogether be eliminated.

Today very careful monitoring is essential to reduce side effects. The minimum dose must be ascertained and this administered over the shortest period.

Looking at all the disadvantages of steroid therapy tends to make one agree with Mr J. P. Stewart, who, as long ago as 1952, made the following remark in his presidential address to the Laryngology section of the Royal Society of Medicine: 'The patient with allergic rhinitis may well find a good linen handkerchief of more lasting comfort than cortisone.'

In addition to the above drugs there are available many that aim to relieve congestion of the bronchi and so help breathing. These are known as 'bronchodilators'.

Bronchodilators work by stimulating that part of the brain that controls breathing and so, by relaxing muscle spasms, open up the air passages into the lungs. Such drugs as adrenaline, ephedrine, sulbutamol and terbutaline act on the 'sympathetic' nerves that control the muscles of the bronchi and so dilate the airways. Others, like atropine, and derivatives of belladonna block the 'parasympathic' nerves that cause the bronchi to constrict. These types of drugs tend to cause discomfort by drying up natural secretions of the airways.

Cromoglycate disodium (INTAL) has been widely used in hayfever and allergic asthma. On administration in powder form it has proved very effective in giving relief. Its side effects are limited and consequently it is widely prescribed. In 1983 the NHS spent five million pounds on this one drug!

When one looks at the various drug therapies available, with their various side effects, some of which are quite serious, and also the huge cost to the Health Service, one wonders whether it is the right approach. Today our system of medicine tends to be geared in relieving symptoms and not actually curing the disease. One doctor with similar views wrote to the *Lancet* in October 1983 concluding that 'the emphasis is all on drugs that may suppress but will never cure'. We will see that the use of honey as a natural medicine to treat these diseases actually *cures* them and carries with it no risk of side effects. However, before we look into the treatment with honey, let us examine an alternative approach to treating hayfever, that of preventing the allergens reaching the sensitive tissues of the nose and eyes.

Prevention of Hayfever

Hayfever has posed a major challenge to physicians ever since it was first described in the early part of the nineteenth century. One obvious means of preventing it is to create a physical barrier between the respiratory tract and the outside world. Many ingenious contraptions have been devised to prevent pollen reaching the sensitive mucous membranes. A casual glance through the pages of the *British Medical Journal* over the last hundred years reveals an assortment of curious and sometimes ingenious contraptions designed to aid the hayfever sufferer. For instance, a black silk nose-bag packed with cotton wool and attached to the nose by way of elastic around the ears was frequently worn by sufferers in late Victorian times. Another device was a face mask consisting of three thicknesses of the finest butter cloth which completely covered the nose and mouth. Various strange devices were used to block the lacrymal ducts, or the nostrils. For those who had the money, and time, a long sea voyage was recommended. In another instance patients were told to adopt a mode of life contained within specially constructed air-filtered rooms.

Most of these efforts were futile and soon found to be so. It was some time early this century that a 'Hayfever Club' was instigated, with members spending the hayfever season comfortably installed on the island of Heligoland. But for those who had occupations to follow, treatment was either a choice of the cumbersome barrier methods or some form of drug treatment.

In the *Sunday Times* of 13 June 1982 a Mr Richard Hinchcliffe announced to the world his invention of the 'Hincherton Hayfever Helmet'. Essentially this was a large perspex dome connected to a battery-driven filtering system. Retailing at about fifty pounds this was the twentieth century version of the spring-clips and nose-bags so much recommended a century earlier.

Thus the management of hayfever had gone full circle revealing that modern medicine had not been able to find an effective cure for this distressing complaint. However, one must admire the persistence of the medical profession. If one reads through the *British Medical Journal* from the late 1870's until the early 1950's, when antihistamines were first introduced, one discovers a treasure house of bizarre and long-forgotten remedies including injections of belladonna, arsenic, morphine, calcium chloride, alchohol, or tuberculin. Face washes with a variety of solutions were recommended including, lemon juice, rain water, salicylic acid and in one instance even cyanide. Fascinating inhalations were also recommended including such substances as phenol, oil of turpentine and specially formulated snuff. Burning cannabis resin or touch paper in the bedroom at night was also advocated.

On another occasion, fuming nitric acid was recommended for direct application to the delicate nasal tissues. One enthusiastic physician even recommended pumping fourteen litres of carbon dioxide into the patient's rectum, one supposes this gave him something else to worry about other than his hayfever! A more dangerous procedure is recorded in the *Journal of the American Medical Association* of 1922, when it was recommended to use radium to irradiate both the nose and eyes of the poor hayfever sufferer. No doubt a more popular remedy was that recommended by an English physician, namely that of drinking spruce beer three times a day — it was certainly less drastic than many of the other forms of treatment.

One concludes that orthodox medicine, during the short time that hayfever has been recognised as a disease, has been unable to find a satisfactory, and safe treatment. It is not surprising, therefore, for disillusioned patients, like Mr Hinchcliffe, to seek relief in adopting what can only be described as ridiculous barrier methods. However, there is one further medical procedure, on which many doctors at present rely, namely, immunotherapy.

Immunotherapy

The theory behind the immunotherapeutic treatment of hayfever and allergic rhinitis is to block the allergic response that occurs after allergens have been inhaled. The simple view is to cause enhanced IgG antibody production at the expense of IgE. This over-production of IgG may be thought of as effectively removing the troublesome allergen from the circulation.

Immunotherapy, has variously been referred to as 'desensitization' or 'hyposensitization'. It usually involves the doctor giving the patient a series of injections that contain gradually increasing doses of allergen. The first of these injections contains so little of the allergen as to be almost negligible; with subsequent injections the dosage is gradually increased.

Unfortunately, as in other walks of life, medicine is influenced by whatever theory, or treatment, is fashionable at any particular time. After Pasteur and Koch it was fashionable to think of all diseases in terms of micro-organisms. Indeed the work of Blackley, on the role of pollen in hayfever, was completely ignored for more than thirty years, because people could only think of it as being caused by a specific bacterium. So too with immunology, which because of its great success has been seen to have the solution for all diseases. Thus, in the early days of immunological science, the excitement that the great developments engendered, created an environment that made scientists think that even hayfever could be treated immunologically.

The world centre for immunology during the early part of this century was Sir Almroth Wright's department at St Mary's Hospital, London. It was here in 1907 that Dr Leonard Noon devised the immunotherapeutic treatment for hayfever. In Wright's inoculation department it seemed perfectly logical that every disease could be treated by injecting antigens.

Noon's sister happened to be a botanist and it was with her assistance that the grass pollens were collected. Extracts were prepared and a procedure consisting of fifty-four desensitizing injections instigated.

It was a long drawn-out procedure and as such was expensive from the point of view of a doctor's time. Consequently, patients were instructed to self-inoculate. The first trials took place in the summer of 1911 and within a short period of time the whole procedure was adopted as satisfactory and safe. This procedure, with minor change, has continued ever since. It is, however, not without its problems. Many doctors today consider it to be unsafe, and many patients would rather continue to suffer from the illness than take this treatment.

In the early days self-inoculation was encouraged. Even young children were instructed on how to inoculate themselves with the pollen extract. Dr John Freeman, a colleague of Sir Alexander Fleming, wrote in his book *Hayfever, a Key to the Allergic Disorders*, published in 1950: '(self-inoculation) is found to be quite practicable for intelligent children over 8 years of age . . .' It is difficult to read these words without having one's faith in the medical profession profoundly shaken. As immunotherapy is not completely safe, for patients — particularly children — to have been encouraged to inject themselves at home is nothing short of irresponsible. Particularly in the light of the fact that a safe, and effective, treatment for hayfever, using honey, was completely ignored simply because it was a 'traditional' or 'folk' remedy.

No doubt it can be argued that the small number of deaths that did occur as a result of the injections were small in comparison to the number of people treated. But surely *one* unnecessary death is too many when we are dealing with a condition, namely, hayfever which is not life-threatening.

The great risk from using immunotherapy arises from the possibility of inducing an anaphylactic shock which frequently is fatal. Any one of Noon's fifty-four self-administered injections could have had a fatal outcome. One wonders how many patients actually have died from this treatment over the years. No-one will ever know. Neither Noon, nor Freeman, could claim ignorance of this very real danger.

An early warning was published in the September issue of the *Journal of the American Medical Association* for the year 1920. In this article Dr W. Walter described how a previously safe injection of pollen extract induced anaphylaxis in one of his patients, thus:

> Mr A B aged 40 had an injection of pollen extract — within 10 seconds there was violent sneezing which quickly developed into paroxysms. In about 5 minutes the patient was in a profound anaphylactic shock. The pulse was hardly palpable and the patient was cyanotic . . .

Unnecessary deaths, particularly among young people, still occur today. A few case-histories from the pages of the *British Medical Journal* for September 1980 will vouch for this fact:

1. An otherwise healthy nineteen-year-old girl attended a Southampton GP for her fourteenth injection of pollen extract. Within five minutes of receiving the injection she began to wheeze and five minutes later she was dead.
2. A twenty-four-year-old male patient attended his Plymouth GP for his fifteenth injection of pollen extract. Within an hour of his receiving it he died in the surgery.

There are several reasons for these fatalities. One problem with some of the desensitization reagents is the variation in potency that exists between different batches, and the loss in potency that occurs during storage in the doctor's surgery. Even though more intensely purified allergens are now available compared to when the technique was first introduced there still exist considerable problems.

In October 1980 Dr Pamela Ewan, herself of the department of

Immunology, St Mary's Hospital, described immunotherapy with pollen extracts as 'potentially dangerous and often ineffective'. Many other doctors and consultants share this view, here are a few of their comments:

> 'For many years I have had desensitization treatment without noticeable benefit.'
>
> A General Practitioner (*BMJ* August 1979)

> 'How far grass pollen vaccines help remains uncertain.'
>
> A London consultant (*BMJ* November 1982)

> 'My hayfever has now lasted for 40 years . . . the results of desensitization seemed to me disappointing.'
>
> A Birmingham consultant (*BMJ* July 1979)

> 'The duration of benefit (from pollen vaccines) is unknown.'
>
> A consultant (*BMJ* September 1981)

Honey Therapy

The use of honey in the treatment of hayfever has a long and successful record. Unlike all the other therapies it is completely harmless with no possible side effects. Let us look at how the idea developed.

It had been known for a great many years that if cows eat grass tops they secrete pollen in their milk. Some hayfever sufferers may get an attack following ingestion of milk containing grass pollen. Possibly this could account for malaise of the English philosopher Robert Burton who wrote in 1651 in his book *The Anatomy of Melancholy* that 'all that comes from milk increases melancholy'.

The fact that pollen could be ingested and pass through the digestive tract and be secreted by way of body fluids must have suggested to early investigators that it might be possible to immunize against the allergens in pollen by its oral ingestion. In the 1920's Drs Touart, Clock, Rubenstone and Scheppegell working in New York developed a method of treating hayfever by just this method. Other methods involving the intranasal application of pollen were tried. But it was a natural progression of these approaches to adopt the long known folk remedy involving the ingestion of honey, which if pure, and preferably comb honey, was rich in pollen. In May 1937 an article on this treatment appeared in the *Transactions of the Association of Military Surgeons* of the USA written by Captain George D. McGrew of the US Army. He wrote:

> Among the many home remedies for the treatment of hayfever which were brought up in discussions with the afflicted, one alone seemed of real value. Several individuals stated that in the past year, or two, they had received varying degrees of relief from symptoms by the eating of honey produced in their vicinity and particularly from the chewing of the comb wax. It was reasonable to infer from this that the benefit received was probably from the oral extraction of the pollen in the honey and wax.

Major Seymour Schwartz of the US Medical Corps referred to the results as 'almost sensational'.

This treatment, however, had been well known in folk medicine and amongst beekeepers for a long time. It was further brought to a wider audience in the book *Folk Medicine* by Dr D. C Jarvis, first published in 1958. Dr Jarvis recommended chewing one teaspoonful of honeycomb, three times a day, commencing at least four months before the hayfever season begins. Furthermore he drew attention to the observation that honey cappings, being richer in pollen, were more effective.

Since that time various modifications of this simple treatment have been promulgated by different authors, and there are now many well documented case-histories of sufferers being completely cured.

Some authors specify that the honey must be locally produced, and in some cases go so far as to state that it must be obtained within a ten mile radius of the patient's home. This does seem unlikely to be so, for two reasons. Firstly, as pollen is blown by the wind over considerable distances, the pollen causing hayfever in a patient need not have originated in his locality. Secondly, if a patient, by eating locally produced honey were to protect himself against local pollens, what would happen if he travelled outside the specified area? Would he have an attack of hayfever? If so, the honey treatment could not be considered to be in any way a cure.

Let us now look at possible explanations regarding how possibly the honey treatment might work. It seems logical that the pollen in the honey is the active ingredient. But this immediately raises a problem because in Britain most sufferers of hayfever are allergic to grass pollens which are rarely found in honey.

It might be possible that the allergens in grass pollen have similar structures to those present in the normal floral pollen found in honey. Thus antibodies produced in patients who have eaten honey pollen might 'cross-react' with the pollen causing the hayfever. To appreciate how antibodies are produced following oral ingestion of pollen we need to account for the lack of destruction of these allergens on entering the digestive tract. In other words, how do they reach the bloodstream without being affected or altered in any way? To do this we need to appreciate the unique anatomy of pollen. Pollen grains consist of an outside shell made of the virtually indestructable material known as sporopollenin. It is this rigid material that enables pollen to remain unaltered for thousands of years in peat bogs and so on. Within this shell are small pores that lead to the interior where the bulk of the allergens are located. Diffusion is slow from both within to the outside and from the outside to within. Thus pollen entering the digestive tract would be little affected by the presence of digestive enzymes which would have difficulty diffusing into the interior of the pollen grain. Thus the large bulk of allergens within a pollen grain would reach the intestinal tract more or less unaltered. Here they could be transported from the lumen epithelial cells into the bloodstream. In experiments with dogs that have been fed pollen in milk, intact pollen grains have been found in the bloodstream two hours after ingestion. Once pollen is in the bloodstream allergens would slowly diffuse out of the sporopollenin shell and induce the gradual build-up of specific antibodies.

Alternatively, there could be a much more complex explanation that does not involve the production of antibodies in response to specific pollen allergens. This is suggested by the fact that other allergies, including allergic asthma, may be treated successfully with comb honey. These observations were made by Dr William Peterson of the Sugg Clinic in Ada, Oklahoma and published in the *American Bee Journal* in 1969. Dr Peterson, an allergist, found that he could successfully treat patients having a wide variety of different allergies, including bronchial asthma, with pure honey. His treatment consisted of small daily doses of honey, which he specified must be pure, unprocessed and in particular, unheated.

Dr Peterson's treatment of bronchial asthma using unheated honey was nothing new. Charak, the famous Ayurvedic physician, recommended the use of pure, unheated honey in the treatment of asthma. Also, Sir John Hill in his book *The Virtues of Honey* published in 1759 recommended honey for asthmatic patients. Dr Donald Monro in his *Treatise on Medical and Pharmaceutical Chymistry and the Materia Medica* published in London in the year 1788 gave the following remarkable account of the curative properties of honey:

> The late Dr John Hume, of the Commissioners of the Sick and Hurt of the Royal Navy, was for many years violently afflicted with asthma. Having taken many medicines without receiving any relief, he at last resolved to try the effects of honey. For two or three years he ate some ounces of it daily and got entirely free of his asthma, and likewise of a gravelly complaint which he had long been afflicted with. About two years after he had recovered his health when he was sitting one day in the Office for the Sick and Hurt, a person labouring under a great difficulty of breathing, who looked as if he could not live many days, came to him, and asked him by what means he had been cured of his asthma? Dr Hume told him the particulars of his own case, and mentioned to him the means by which he had found relief. For two years after he heard nothing of this person, who was a stranger to him, and had seemed so bad that he did not imagine that he could have lived many days, and therefore had not even asked him who he was; but at the end of that period, a man seemingly in good health, and decently dressed, came to the Sick and Hurt Office and returned him thanks for his cure, which he assured him had been entirely brought about by the free use of honey.

The fact that honey is an effective means of treatment, not only for hayfever, but for other allergies as well, might suggest that its mode of operation in patients is not a straightforward desensitization. Therefore, could there be another mechanism involving some physiologically active biochemical in the pollen? Pollen is really a remarkable substance, containing innumerable biologically-active biochemicals, many of them as yet uncharacterized. It would be wrong to speculate too freely. What is more justified is to look at what has been definitely found in pollen and go from there.

Rape honey has, for example, been found to contain the steroid brassinolide. The structure of this biochemical is remarkably similar to belomethasone, one of the corticosteroids used to treat allergic asthma. Furthermore, many flavanoids have been discovered in pollen, a number of them bearing a resemblance of the structure of cromoglycate, one of the most successful and widely-used allergy drugs. Could there be other substances, not yet identified, that are more similar to the drugs in current usage? Could some of these biochemicals be more potent than the drugs now used to treat these complaints?

The treatment with honey requires a small quantity to be digested daily over a long period. Such a remedy would be useless in treating an acute attack, but the prolonged and regular ingestion of honey, rich in pollen, could maintain within the body a low 'background' level of these active biochemicals that eventually would eliminate the disease entirely. Thus a low dose of an active biochemical over a very long period of time might be more beneficial than a hefty dosage just when symptoms appear.

An alternative explanation is that the remarkable potency of honey is derived from the small traces of bee venom it contains. This originates from the manner in which honey is processed in the hive by the worker bee, for as soon as the honey in the honeycomb is almost capped she injects a minute trace of venom just beneath the capping. This ensures that the honey remains pure and fresh.

Recent studies by biochemists have shown bee venom to be an extremely complex substance, but what is most relevant has been the discovery that the long-held folk tradition that bee venom may bring relief to some forms of rheumatic disease does indeed have a scientific basis. In particular, one substance present in the venom has been found to have strong anti-inflammatory activity. This substance, when present in honey, would interact with natural pollen grains in such a way that would enable it to pass through the digestive tract in man and be eventually absorbed into the blood. Here it would exert its anti-inflammatory activity, but more importantly it would induce the release of natural corticosteroids. This has been shown to happen in laboratory experiments. Furthermore, there is strong evidence that these natural substances are responsible for the beneficial effects of honey, particularly in conditions such as hayfever and allergic asthma.

In summary therefore, if honey is to be successful in the treatment of hayfever, or other similar allergic diseases then three important conditions must be fulfilled. These are:

1. the honey must be entirely pure and had the minimum of heat processing;
2. it must have a high pollen content, which implies that it has not been filtered. And,
3. that it must be taken in small amounts, regularly over a long period.

CHAPTER 10
Unusual Honeys

Allergy to Honey

Food allergy is now well recognized. However, although allergies to eggs and strawberries are relatively common, allergic reaction to honey is virtually unknown.

When it does occur very small quantities of honey are sufficient to bring a person out in a generalised skin rash. The reason why honey should produce such an allergy is not known for certain, but it is probably a reaction to the pollen it contains. It must be stressed, however, that this type of allergy is extremely rare. Throughout the whole of the literature on honey there are only a few references to it. One instance was mentioned by the entomologist William Kirby (1759–1850) who knew of a woman to whom ordinary honey acted like poison. He mentions symptoms such as nausea and intestinal disturbances characteristic of such an allergy. He also recorded an instance of death following the consumption of honey. Although it is difficult to evaluate the significance of this from the limited details he provided it does, however, seem more likely that this was a case of honey poisoning rather than allergy.

Toxic Honey

Toxic honey has been known to exist since antiquity. There are references in the Old Testament suggesting that some honeys may have unpleasant side reactions, thus: 'Hast thou found honey? eat so much as is sufficient for thee, lest thou be filled therewith and vomit it (Proverbs 27:16) and, 'It is not good to eat much honey . . .' (Proverbs 27:27).

The most famous account of toxic honey is that given by Xenophon in the fourth book of the Anabasis.

In 400 BC Xenophon's army of ten thousand men had reached the area on the Black Sea near Trebizond. The account continues:

> The number of beehives was extraordinary and all the soldiers who ate of the combs lost their senses, vomited and were affected with purging, and none of them were able to stand upright. Those who had eaten only a little behaved as if drunk, and those who had eaten much were like madmen. Others were like persons on the point of death. Consequently they lay on the ground in great numbers as if it had been a defeat. The following day not one of them was found dead, and they recovered their senses about the same hour that they had lost them on the day before. On the third and fourth day they were able to get up and felt as if they had taken medicine.

This account quite clearly points out that the troublesome honey was not wild honey, but honey actually taken from beehives. One may presume that the local people would have later consumed this honey so why was it toxic to Xenophon's men? Probably the explanation is that they had eaten *unripe* honey in which toxins were present. If the honey had been allowed to mature these toxins would have disappeared.

We know today that in parts of Georgia and Florida honey from the yellow jessamine (*Gelsemium sempervirens*) is poisonous only when it is uncapped. An incident was described by F. C. Pellett in 1885 when three children died from eating this honey when it was unripe. Whereas eating the ripe honey was perfectly safe.

Other honeys obtained near Trebizond are also known to be toxic. The honey of Heracleia Pontica further to the west was occasionally known to make those who had eaten it roll on the ground in considerable pain. Colchis, further to the north also produced a toxic honey known as 'maddening honey'. Strabo (60 BC--AD 20) the Greek geographer recorded that Colchian honey was bitter. In more recent times the traveller Evliyá Effendi warned people against eating this honey. He also advised against eating honey of the Erzerum province, thus: '. . . bread and honey are rather to be suspected, for I myself, poor Evliyá, having eaten some honey in the commander's house, became in half an hour so giddy that I thought of throwing myself down from the castle' (von Hammer, *The Travels of Evliyá Effendi* II, p. 119)

The French botanist Joseph Tournefort (1656–1708) attributed the poisonous honey to two species of rhododendron after local people had informed him that the perfume of the flowers caused severe headaches.

The honey from the Trebizond area is probably the most famous but other poisonous honeys are known.

In North America during the autumn of 1790 extensive mortality occurred amongst those who had eaten honey in the neighbourhood of Philadelphia (*American Philosophical Transactions* 1790, v). The American government became so concerned that an inquiry was set up to investigate the incident. This concluded that the honey had been obtained from the mountain laurel (*Kalmia latifolia*). In more recent years this plant has caused similar problems, indeed it has been known for beekeepers to throw hundreds of pounds of honey into rivers and streams if they think their bees have collected nectar from this plant. Furthermore, in certain parts of western North Carolina it is impossible to produce edible honey because of the presence of this plant.

Some people have treated the whole problem of poisonous honey with disbelief. One reason being is that it is very difficult to get the same reaction to the honey in different seasons. (This problem has been apparent since antiquity as Pliny was considerably puzzled by it.) A further difficulty has been identifying the toxic constituent of the honey. For example, a sample of the toxic honey from North Carolina was found to be pure by analysts in Washington, however the County Apiarist after eating a small sample wrote: 'there was a tingling of the fingers and toes as if the circulation had been stopped. Very soon it was difficult to stand. This was followed by a severe headache which lasted a couple of hours.'

According to the Russian writer Z. Gutnikova, poisonous honey is obtained from the leather-leaf plant. This honey is slightly yellow in colour with a somewhat bitter taste and granulates readily. Apparently it is toxic to man but not for bees. When small amounts are eaten, it produces violent headaches, shivering, nausea and vomiting. As little as one teaspoonful is sufficient to lead to delirium and loss of consciousness. In the Khabarovsk region of Russia so-called 'heady honey' is obtained from the marsh tea plant.

Lord Macaulay (1800–1859) in his essay on Milton refers to the melancholy of Dante as: 'resembling that noxious Sardinian soil of which the intense bitterness is said to have been perceptible even in its honey.' Macaulay was wrong in his assumption that it was the bitterness of the soil, for we now know it to be due to the bees collecting nectar from a local variety of wild parsley. Recent investigations have shown the toxin in this honey to be a new type of alkaloid.

In South Africa the missionary Robert Moffat (1795–1883) described coming across a plant of the *Euphorbia* family which produced a poisonous honey. When eaten the honey gave a burning sensation in the throat; and in the Pretoria region it was known as 'Noors honey'.

As mentioned above many of the reports concerning poisonous honey were at first treated with scepticism by scientists. Many even refused to believe the stories that came down from antiquity. Only in recent years have organic chemists performed careful analytical studies on these honeys and confirmed that they indeed do contain toxins.

The first serious study of this problem was described in the *British Medical Journal* of 26 November 1887. Two tins of honey were sent by the Consul at Trebizond to the Pharmaceutical Society of London. Careful examination did indeed establish the honey to be poisonous but because the methods of identification used at that time were inadequate, the toxins could not be recognised. It was not until the 1960's that techniques had developed sufficiently to identify the complex substances present in this honey.

From plants of the *Ericaceae* family the toxins have been found to be terpenoid in nature. They have been called 'grayanotoxins'. So far over 30 different ones have been isolated and identified. Another type of toxin has been found in the honeydew, from the Tutu plant in New Zealand. In this instance the passion-vine hopper *Scolypopa australis* ingests the toxin tutin from the plant and converts it into mellitoxin which is excreted along with the honeydew. This is gathered by the bees and stored with their honey. (See Table 4.)

Conclusion

It must again be emphasized that toxic honey is exceedingly rare and unlikely to be encountered in Britain.

Its significance serves to illustrate the complexity of honey. The fact that minute amounts of plant toxins can be incorporated into honey highlights the likelihood that trace quantities of antimicrobial substances are also likely. This will be discussed in the next chapter.

Table 4

Toxins identified in rare honeys

Name of Toxin	***Source***	***Toxin concentration in honey (parts per million)***
acetylandromedol, (grayanotoxin 1)	Honey from, *Kalmia,* Rhododendron	80–100
tutin (and hyenanchin)	honeydew of *Coriaria arboria* (tutu tree)	20
pyrrolizidine alkaloids (jacobine, jacozine)	Honey from tansy and ragwort (*Senecio jacobaea*)	3
gelsemine	Honey from yellow jessamine (*Gelsemium sempervirens*)	40

CHAPTER 11

The Antibiotic Nature of Honey

We have considered in the previous chapter how honey may occasionally contain substances that are toxic to man. Fortunately, only a very few honeys actually contain these substances that come directly from the plant nectar. The considerable research that has been carried out into toxic honey has revealed how nectar contributes a vast array of chemical substances that eventually go to make up honey. Many of these substances are present in minute concentration and so have no immediately obvious biological role. However, when individually isolated many have been found to have remarkable biological activity. Only a very small number of them have been found to be toxic to man. Unfortunately few of the other substances have attracted the attention of biochemists and so they remain, as yet, uncharacterized.

In chapter three the argument was developed which suggested that for nectar-bearing plants to have evolved, depending as they do upon insect pollination for reproduction, then they must also have developed an armoury of antimicrobial substances. Logically these would be present in the nectar, for this is the attractant for the insects, which are potential vectors of disease.

Consequently nectar is a possible source for new antibiotic substances. But as honey is concentrated nectar it should be a much richer source. This rather simple view is reinforced by the great mass of scientific evidence that points to the presence of antibiotics in honey. Let us now examine firstly the historical and largely circumstantial evidence, and then go on to look at the most significant scientific findings. In addition, some recent clinical observations on the use of honey as an antibiotic will be considered.

Historical Evidence

Since antiquity it has been known that honey is able to prevent bacterial decay. Both the ancient Egyptians and the Greeks used honey to embalm their dead. We know from history that after Alexander the Great's death, his body was returned for burial in Macedonia immersed in honey. The traveller Evilyà Effendi gave an account of how the people of Abaza would bury their dead: 'they would put the body into a wooden coffin which they would nail on the branches of some high tree and make a hole in it near the head. Bees would enter and make honey, entirely wrapping the body up in it.'

The knowledge that honey could prevent the dead decaying must have suggested to primitive people that honey could also stop wounds becoming putrid. So we find that the ancient Egyptians depended almost entirely on the effectiveness of honey for the management of wounds. Presumably this same idea occurred to other peoples for we find that in Ayurvedic Medicine the same dependence upon honey for the treatment of wounds. According to Dr C. Dwarakanath, a Principal of the Ayurvedic College in Mysore, honey is used today, and has been for the past two thousand years, in Ayurvedic medicine for this purpose.

The most celebrated physician of antiquity, Hippocrates (460–377 BC) who collected together many of the traditional treatments, from the early history of medicine, wrote of honey: 'It causes heat, cleans sores, and ulcers, softens hard ulcers of the lips, heals carbuncles and running sores. Furthermore, it is known that he used honey regularly in his medical practice. It is interesting to note that for centuries after his death, honey, from his island of Cos, was collected and used to treat thrush in nursing mothers.

Several hundred years later Pliny (AD 23–79) carried out a similar survey of traditional remedies. His work, however, was not confined to medicine. The *Historia Naturalis* is a mammoth work containing a vast amount of information on almost every topic. Only one part is concerned with folk remedies. Some of these treatments have been 'rediscovered', in recent times, and developed into modern drugs.

One such example is ephedrine, a drug that has been widely used in modern medicine, and yet Pliny described its isolation from the plant he called *Ephedron (Ephedra nebrodensis)* long before its modern rediscovery.

This vividly illustrates the value of folk medicine for us today. Although the scientific understanding of disease has progressed at a tremendous pace throughout the last hundred years, we should not ignore much of the empirical knowledge gained by our ancestors.

Honey was frequently mentioned and recommended by Pliny. In particular he described it as 'being applied on wool to old sores'. He also points out its virtue in the treatment of oral abscesses.

In ancient Russian medical books honey is repeatedly recommended for 'fetid wounds'. An early English manuscript, the eleventh-century *Leechbook of Bald*, advises the treatment of 'foul' wounds and amputations with honey. In the Middle Ages honey was extensively used in the form of ointments and plasters for boils, wounds, burns and ulcers. All over the Far East honey has been used in folk medicine as a cure for boils. Mixed with soap and applied to the boil it rapidly brings it to a head and draws out all the pus.

Thus throughout a large part of man's history honey has been relied upon as a safe and effective antibiotic. Let us now look at some recent clinical observations.

Clinical Observations

Some of the earliest clinical observations on the use of honey in the treatment of wounds comes from veterinary science. Zaiss, working in Germany in 1934, published the results of his extensive experience in using honey to treat thousands of wounds in animals. He found that honey, in comparison to other medicants available at that time, was very much superior. He stressed, however, that the honey had to be freshly obtained from the comb and that it must not have been heated. The following year Dr Zaiss, together with his co-worker Dr Lühr, published further evidence as to the highly effective nature of honey in wound management.

These findings were independently confirmed by Dr M. Marienburg of Hannover, in 1939.

As war approached the need to find an effective treatment for wounds intensified. Dr W. Müller investigated the use of honey in the treatment of mustard gas lesions in experimental rabbits. This researcher was considerably impressed with his findings. Not only was there an indication of a shortening of the healing period but that the incidence of secondary infections was reduced.

It was not only in the West that there was interest in the use of honey in wound treatment. In 1944, Dr K. L. Yang, writing in the journal *Chinese Medicine* described how an ointment consisting of four parts of honey, to one part of lard, was used in the traditional medicine of China. He reported that this ointment was highly effective in the management of small wounds and ulcers. In particular he found it very useful in the treatment of dirty and infected wounds when it had a positive cleansing effect. Furthermore, Dr Yang found that honey led to a subsidence of inflammation and stimulated tissue regrowth. He concluded that honey was generally well tolerated, basically harmless and very effective.

In Russia, the Soviet surgeon Dr Y. Krinitsky used a mixture of honey and cod-liver oil, as an ointment for festering wounds. He found that the mixture had a soothing effect and, despite its stickiness, the dressings did not adhere to the wounds. Dr Krinitsky recorded success rates of more than ninety per cent and was led to the view that honey actually accelerated the wound healing process.

During World War II Professor S. Smirnov of the Tomsk Medical Institute applied honey to bullet wounds and found that it stimulated tissue regeneration, particularly in sluggishly healing wounds.

Hippocrates had observed that honey was particularly useful in the treatment of oral wounds. This was confirmed by Russian surgeons. N. Yoirish in his book *Curative Properties of Honey* published in Moscow in 1959, described a sixty-three-year-old patient who, after resection of the larynx for removal of a malignant tumour, was treated with honey. The patient's wound quickly healed and ten years afterwards he was still well and actively working.

In 1953, Dr M. D. Quadratullah, writing in the *Karachi Medical Journal*, urged the wider therapeutic use of honey, particularly in underdeveloped countries. However, he stressed that only pure, unprocessed honey was useful medically.

The use of honey in wound management following major surgery has been investigated in this country by the late Michael Bulman, one time consultant surgeon at the Norfolk Hospital at Norwich. Writing in the *Middlesex Hospital Journal* in 1955, he described how he and his staff had used honey in cases of vulvectomy and radical surgery of the breast. He concluded:

> Having started with a measure of scepticism on my own part and that of my staff, all those who have seen the effects of honey dressings have become convinced of their value.
>
> 'I have every reason to think that this very simple substance provides one answer to the problem of the treatment of many infected wounds.'

> 'The advantages claimed for it are that it is non-irritating, non-toxic, self-sterile, bactericidal, nutritive, cheap and, above all, effective.

Further remarkable successes have been recorded by Drs Cavanagh, Beasley and Ostapowicz in the *Journal Obstetrics and Gynaecology* (British Commonwealth) of 1970. They studied twelve patients recovering from radical surgery for carcinoma of the vulva. They applied pure honey directly to the wounds and observed rapid healing. Their conclusion was that treatment with honey was far more efficacious than conventional treatment with expensive antibiotics. Furthermore, they reported *in vitro* studies on the bactericidal activity of honey towards a wide range of micro-organisms.

Another surgeon to prove the efficiency of honey was Robert Blomfield who wrote an article in the *Journal of the American Medical Association*, in May 1973, commenting: 'I have found that (honey) when applied every two, or three days, under a dry dressing, promotes the healing of ulcers and burns better than any other local application I have used before.' More recently, Mr P. J. Armon, formerly consultant gynaecologist at the Christian Medical Centre, Kilimanjaro, Tanzania, writing in the journal *Tropical Doctor* for April 1980, outlined his considerable experience with honey in the treatment of wounds. Several case histories illustrating the miraculous properties of honey were given:

1. A twenty-five-year-old woman had a massive bedsore that exposed the bone. A thin layer of pure honey was applied and covered with a dry dressing. Although surgical closure of the wound was planned, this was subsequently found to be unnecessary as the wound closed of its own accord. The patient recovered completely.

2. A twenty-year-old woman who has a grossly infected laparotomy wound failed to respond to antibiotic therapy. Pus was discharging from the wound and vagina. Honey on clean dressings was applied and within two weeks the wound had completely healed without recourse to antibiotics.

Dr Armon concluded that wounds became bacteriologically sterile on the application of honey, which he emphasized was the fresh, locally-produced variety. Furthermore, he found that honey promoted rapid growth of granulation tissue and speeded up the healing process.

From the above accounts there is ample clinical evidence of the beneficial properties of honey. The obvious question to follow is 'Why isn't honey used more by the medical profession?' There are several possible reasons. Firstly, the antibiotics we have in use today are forcefully marketed to doctors and hospitals by very powerful multinational drug companies. These drug companies, because of their extensive advertising, influence the policy of medical journals and, what is more important, the type of research carried on in our universities. Their interest in a particular drug is centred on one thing, namely money. To get money from a drug it must be patentable. Honey is not a patentable substance so therefore no pharmaceutical company is going to invest a considerable amount of money in organising clinical testing of a product they cannot patent. Without controlled clinical trials the medical profession is unimpressed.

It is pertinent to point out that the greatest interest in honey as a natural medicine is in the USSR and other Eastern European countries where medicine is organised rather differently.

Scientific Evidence

Let us now consider the scientific evidence for the presence of antibiotics in honey. This must be looked at in its historical context.

In the early decades of this century there was much concern over the spread of infectious diseases by foods. It was well appreciated that milk was a carrier of several diseases including tuberculosis, which at that time was a major problem.

Honey was rarely considered to present such a hazard. But one day Dr W. G. Sackett, a bacteriologist at the Colorado Agricultural College, observed honey-bees crawling over some excrement and he became convinced that these creatures transmitted disease by way of their honey to man. He therefore initiated some tests to discover how long various disease organisms would survive in honey. To begin with he looked at the organism that causes dysentry to man. To his surprise he discovered that rather than the honey serving as a medium to spread the germs, it actually killed them. Consequently Dr Sackett completely changed his views and came to believe that honey, rather than being a possible carrier of disease, was a potent antibiotic.

More recent studies have confirmed Dr Sackett's views and have vindicated both honey and the honey-bee. The honey-bee in fact has been shown to be a very clean insect. If, for example, one is killed and its body dipped in culture medium, bacteria rarely grow out from it. This does not imply that honey-bees are sterile, for they have a rich intestinal bacterial flora, rather it indicates that within their tissues there are potent antibacterial substances. If so, honey must also contain them, in addition to the antibiotic substances from the plant nectar. Furthermore, honey within the hive is intimately associated with propolis, a substance made by bees from gum exuded from the buds and stems of trees. Propolis has long been recognized as a powerful antibiotic and is widely used as such in Eastern European countries.

Honey also has the unique ability to maintain a sterile environment on account of its extremely hypertonic nature. This tends to abstract water from bacterial cells so leading to their dehydration and death. Dr A. P. Sturtevant, working at the United States Bureau of Entomology in Washington D.C., showed that the organism causing dysentry in man could not survive longer than forty-eight hours when placed in honey. He also discovered that those bacteria that caused broncho-pneumonia and typhoid were similarly destroyed.

Long before the potential usefulness of penicillin was recognized, honey was demonstrated to have antibiotic properties and attracted considerable interest. In 1934 Dr L. Bahr found after doing experiments on white mice that honey could protect them from infection with typhoid bacteria. Attempts to isolate the active substance from honey were fraught with difficulty, as later proved to be so with penicillin. However, in 1937 a paper appeared in the journal *Z. Hyg, Infektkrankl* by a group of German workers who reported isolating from honey an antibiotic to which they gave the name 'inhibine'. This substance was very active and even retained its activity at high dilutions. The substance was both heat and light sensitive and so they could not isolate sufficient of it for chemical characterization. These findings were confirmed in 1938 by Dr M. Prica who found that the bacteriocidal activity of inhibine was towards both gram-positive and gram-negative bacteria.

During the World War II and in the years shortly after, penicillin and related antibiotics occupied the attention of most investigators. However, there were still occasional references in the scientific literature to honey. In 1950 a report appeared by Dr Franz Pothman, of the Institute of Medicine in Dusseldorf, who demonstrated that honey could inhibit the growth of tubercle bacilli. Few other studies were reported until 1962 when workers in the United States proposed that the active substance in honey 'inhibine' was nothing other than hydrogen peroxide.

That hydrogen peroxide was present in honey was nothing new. But these workers proposed that the enzyme glucose oxidase reacted with glucose in the honey producing hydrogen peroxide and gluconic acid. What was new was the concept that the long sought after antibiotic in honey was merely hydrogen peroxide — a cheap and readily available germicide.

This explanation was readily accepted and remains so to this day. I dispute this view completely and maintain that there were other reasons why this view was so conveniently promulgated and readily accepted.

To understand this we must look back to the period of the late 1950's and early 1960's. It was a period of increasing wealth and prosperity in the Western world. World War II had been over for more than a decade and most Western countries were becoming increasingly affluent. People began to have considerably more leisure time and had money to spend on luxuries. Many working people started to take a greater interest in their health. The implication being that they took a greater interest in the food they ate. This is reflected in the upsurge in the health food industry that occurred at this time. This industry grew from nothing shortly after the war, to an industry having an annual turnover of £150 million today. (In the United States the annual turnover is estimated to be around £7000 million!)

Honey therefore began to be marketed as a prime health food and sales of it began to increase. This, however, was not matched by a corresponding increase in home-produced honey, as following the war beekeeping had drastically declined in Britain. This decline was not particularly in the number of small beekeepers but more significantly, from a honey production point of view, in the number of large concerns. It became necessary to import huge quantities of honey into Britain to make up this shortfall in home production. Soon many of the honey packers found that it was far more profitable to deal directly with imported honey rather than be concerned with the unpredictable business of dealing with local honey. Several of the new packing companies were actually set up from what were previously bee farming operations.

The main problem with imported honey however was that it usually arrived in Britain in a granulated form. In order to pack it into jars it was necessary to heat it in order to render it liquid. As we have already discussed, heating honey, ever since the time of the ancient Egyptians, was known to destroy its health-giving properties. How could honey therefore be marketed as a prime health food, if its health-giving properties had been destroyed, in the packing operation?

This was a crucial moment for the honey trade. It was just at this time (1962) that the evidence for the antibiotic in honey to be identified as hydrogen peroxide was published. The significance of this being that it enabled the honey trade to justify its practice of heating honey. They were able to dismiss all the historical and traditional evidence as being due to hydrogen peroxide — a cheap and commonly available germicide. Their view being that if it were simply hydrogen peroxide that was the antibiotic then it was perfectly all right to continue heating the honey during their packing process. Furthermore, the imported product, that had been heated, could be passed off as equivalent to home-produced honey from a nutritional point of view. After all it could no longer be considered to be a medicine; or could it?

This is the situation today, and few people have questioned the validity of the 'inhibine' concept.

Yet, even someone having only a meagre scientific background, should be able to see through the hydrogen peroxide concept for what it really is — utter nonsense. Let us look at the reasons for this. To do so we need to appreciate a little of the chemistry of hydrogen peroxide.

As we have mentioned above, hydrogen peroxide is a germicide. It destroys germs because it is a powerful oxidising agent. This is common knowledge, for it has been used for generations for bleaching, particularly hair. Hydrogen peroxide is now extensively used in washing powder detergents. Their success however is limited by one substance, namely the enzyme catalase. Catalase is present in all biological material and its function is to destroy hydrogen peroxide.

The detergent industry has done extensive research in the search for an inhibitor of catalase action which would enhance the effectiveness of their peroxide-based washing powders. But due to the ubiquitous nature of catalase they have so far failed.

The enzyme catalase is one of the most active enzymes known to man. It is so active that one molecule of it can destroy over two million molecules of hydrogen peroxide, in a fraction of a second. As all cells contain catalase it is easy to appreciate how a minute trace of biological material, blood for instance, amongst the week's laundry, is sufficient to reduce the effectiveness of the washing powder added to the wash.

Honey also contains the enzyme catalase. This is derived from the nectar of plants, which are particularly rich in this enzyme. Although in pure honey, because of its viscous nature, the enzyme will react only slowly, as soon as the honey becomes diluted, on application to a wound for example, reaction will be almost instantaneous. This would destroy all the hydrogen peroxide, none would remain, so therefore how can the hydrogen peroxide be the antibiotic in honey? In my view hydrogen peroxide is neither 'inhibine', nor the antibiotic in honey. There must therefore be some other substance present in honey that gives it its antibiotic activity. So far, this material has not been identified but it is likely to be heat sensitive and so would be absent in mass-produced honey.

Conclusion

Modern medicine tends to rely on antibiotics to treat disease when it has reached an acute stage. It seems more logical however to prevent infection or, at least, arrest it in its early stages. Prevention may be achieved by building up the body's own ability to fight infection before it has got a significant hold.

Good nutrition and emotional stability are vitally important factors that influence the body's defences. Honey may be another. For if it contains minute amounts of an, as yet, unidentified antibiotic substance, a daily intake of it will provide a background level of this substance which could assist the body to stave off infection. There is considerable evidence that those people who do take fresh honey as part of their daily diet are healthier than others who do not. This will be discussed in detail in the next chapter. One thing is certain, a small daily dose of pure home-produced honey can do no harm!

CHAPTER 12
Honey and Longevity?

It is both well known and generally accepted that beekeepers tend to live longer than other people. In Russia where beekeeping has been valued more so than probably in any other country, there exists considerable evidence to support this view. As long ago as the twelfth century the first Russian woman physician Eupraxia-Zoe in a treatise, written in Greek, recommended eating honey to promote health and long life. In more recent times many accounts have appeared in the Soviet literature describing people who have lived to exceptional age, all of whom have been beekeepers or regular consumers of honey. Indeed the Russians have recently issued a commemorative postage stamp in honour of one of these beekeepers who lived to be over 120 years. In his book *Beekeeping for Village Schoolmasters* A. Zubarev tells of a woman living in the village of Nazyi on the Ladoga canal who lived to be 110 years of age and maintained a diet largely of honey. Yoirish in his book *Curative Properties of Honey* describes how he surveyed a large number of centenarians as to their dietary habits and found a consistent common factor in that they all ate honey regularly.

In other cultures there are also similar beliefs in the role honey may have in ensuring longevity. In ancient Indian medicine, for example, the Ayur-Veda advises that human life may be prolonged if a certain diet is adhered to and a principal component of this diet is honey. Dr Bhatia of the Central Food Research Institute of Mysore in India has concluded: 'the beneficial effects of honey cannot be dismissed till they are disproved. We cannot obviously fail to take note of the many centenarians on record, that have been beekeepers and users of honey as a substantial part of their diet.'

Even the most sceptical has to admit that there is almost overwhelming tradition from history behind the belief that when honey is habitually eaten longevity is the result. Pythagoras is believed to have lived on a diet consisting of bread and honey. He died at ninety. One of his followers, Apollonius, who maintained the same diet is believed to have lived to well over a century. Hippocrates is also believed to have eaten honey regularly and to have lived to be over 107 years. Many of the Romans also maintained that health and long life were to be achieved by eating pure honey. The physician Galen in his work *De Sanitate Tuenda* recorded the case histories of two very old men, Telephus and Antiochus, noting that they maintained a very simple diet in which the best raw honey was a major feature.

In all the above records there is the common feature that the honey consumed has been frequently referred to as 'raw', meaning, in effect, that it has been comb honey. This implies that the honey has not been processed, in particular, it has not been heated, nor had its pollen removed. This honey is quite different from what the consumer today is offered in supermarkets. But could fresh, unprocessed honey really have this effect, or is it all folklore? To do controlled experiments with people would be impossible. Several generations would be needed before any results could be secured. Who would fund such research? Indeed, how many scientists would be prepared to carry out experiments, the results of which they would probably not be around to see?

To solve this problem two approaches are possible. Firstly, a careful examination of historical records of proven longevity in people could indicate some common factor. This, however, is notoriously unreliable simply because old people tend to attribute their great age to a wide variety of unassociated factors. In particular, as their memories are on the whole unreliable, they might say they have eaten a particular food over a long period of time which in fact they have not. However, it is much easier to establish how long a person has kept bees and it is a good assumption that that person has eaten his own honey. This association, therefore, could carry more weight than others.

A much more promising approach is to carry out experiments on animals. In fact some remarkable experiments have been reported. These show that not only is longevity possible, but that it is also accompanied by enhanced virility in the male, and fertility in the female.

These experiments have been carried out with butterflies of the neotropical genus *Heliconius*, and published by Dr Lawrence Gilbert of the University of Texas, in the *Proceedings of the National Academy of Sciences* of the USA, in June 1972. Dr Gilbert actually did not use honey in his experiments but a mixture of pollen and nectar. This is of course equivalent to pure unprocessed honey and so it is perfectly valid to make the extrapolation of his findings to imply similar effects with honey. Dr Gilbert found that it was the presence of pollen that was most significant. For normal butterflies live only a matter of weeks, whereas *Heliconius ethilla*, when fed pollen and nectar, lived for as long as six months. Dr Gilbert concluded that it was the nutrients in the pollen that enabled these butterflies to live to this exceptional age. If the pollen was removed from their diet they no longer had the same life span.

A further remarkable finding was the enhanced fertility of the butterflies. Those females fed a diet of pollen and nectar laid five times as many eggs as those fed nectar alone. Furthermore, old specimens of five months old still laid eggs at the same rate as when young, whereas those butterflies not fed pollen laid eggs for only the first few days of adult life. Dr Gilbert also noticed that the males also were able to maintain sexual activity throughout their long life. This did not happen with the control group. Dr Gilbert concluded that this species of butterfly was able to extract from the pollen certain nutrients enabling it to go on living to this exceptional age.

Could these experiments have significance in our discussion as to the role of honey in longevity in man? I think so, for although they relate to feeding pollen and nectar, this is really identical with honey, in particular honey that is fresh, unprocessed, unheated, and which has not had its pollen removed. This is precisely the material that throughout history has been associated with records in man of both longevity and fertility. Could this be mere coincidence?

One could of course point out that these experiments on butterflies are irrelevant to man and that the historical evidence associating honey consumption with longevity is misleading. For example, is the association more likely to be that of beekeeping and longevity, rather than that of actual honey consumption? It is true beekeepers tend to live sober lives, generally in tranquil country areas, so could it be their overall life style? Alternatively one could point to the fact that beekeeping in general attracts a particular type of personality. As beekeeping is largely a solitary occupation many beekeepers tend to be rather introverted. Many would be described as 'loners'. Indeed, there are some beekeepers who prefer the company of bees to people. This must have been so throughout history as Cicero and Pliny record one Hyliscus who quit human society to live amongst bees.

As bees are much more predictable than humans, could a life spent largely amongst bees be considerably less stressful than one managing people? I think it probably could be. Thus it could be that the beekeeping personality tends to longevity rather than his consumption of honey. One drawback of this argument is that it fails to account for the longevity of those who have consumed honey but have not been beekeepers.

One is forced to reach the conclusion that there is considerable evidence that a regular consumption of honey is likely to promote longevity but one is forced to admit there are clearly other factors involved which might override its significance. However, we can be certain about one thing and that is honey can do no harm. So let us now turn our attention away from the complex area of longevity to see if the consumption of honey can play any significant role in preventing premature death.

One of the main causes of premature death in man in the world today is cancer. It is curious, but here again there is widespread belief that beekeepers are less prone to cancer than the rest of the population. What is the origin of this concept and is there any truth in it? If there is how can it be accounted for?

In fact it does seem to have some scientific basis for recent epidemiological surveys seem to give it support. In particular a survey recently carried out in the Department of Biostatistics and Epidemiology at the Sidney Farber Cancer Institute in the United States provides ample evidence in support of this idea. In this survey the causes of death of 580 beekeepers who died between 1950 and 1978 were examined and compared with a comparable group of the general population. It was found that there were significantly less cases of malignancy amongst the beekeepers than the other group.

Having shown there is a significant difference, how can it be explained? Is it, for instance, to do with the regular consumption of honey, or is it some other factor related to beekeeping? Tradition has it that it is related to the incidence of bee stings.

What we must now ask is, could it be possible that bee stings are able to affect a beekeeper in some way, so as to delay, or possibly inhibit the development of cancer? I believe it might be so and can think of a number of possible explanations. But firstly, for those who may not have been stung by a bee, it might be instructive for me to relate how the body normally reacts to such an event. As a beekeeper I have been frequently stung and I have made careful notes as to how the body reacts.

To begin with, like many other novice beekeepers, I had a fear of being sensitive to bee stings. As the press normally makes a lot of fuss if a beekeeper dies from a single sting, many beginners have similar apprehensions. However, once one gets into the activity and has received many stings one gets it into proportion and treats stings as mere inconveniences.

Let us take, for example, a sting on the hand. There is of course the immediate sensation of pain, but this quickly subsides and one is left with a small red area of skin. However, within an hour one begins to feel a slight aching of the finger joints. I believe this to be due to the actual movement of white blood cells towards the position of the injury. Slowly the whole area begins to swell up and within about twelve hours it is fully swollen. Then almost exactly forty-eight hours after the sting the redness and swelling completely goes away.

What I have described are the immediate effects, but what are the long-term effects of a bee sting? As far as I know this has not been investigated, as most authorities consider only the immediate effects. But such a traumatic event must have significant long-term effects on the body's immune system. There is, of course, the development of an immunity to the bee venom itself, but as to what other effects it has, no-one knows. I believe there must be significant long-term effects on the immune system for it has been known for centuries that bee stings can prevent, and even cure, certain rheumatic diseases.

It is generally accepted that as one ages the body's immune system becomes less efficient. Indeed, one widely accepted view as to the origin of cancer is to consider that the immune system has declined to destroy the original malignant cell that originated the particular cancer. This view is strengthened by the findings from studying AIDS victims who, because of their disease, have a weak immune system and so are accordingly very susceptible to the development of certain cancers.

Could it be, therefore, that the regular and frequent bee stings received by beekeepers are a continual challenge to their immune systems? Does it keep their defences in prime condition? Although one can argue that beekeepers gain immunity to bee venom itself this, in fact, is never complete as the strain of bee is continually changing in the average apiary, and all the different varieties of bee will have slightly differing venom. This being in effect a continual challenge to the beekeeper's immune system.

A further possibility is that there is a build-up of immunity against the enzyme hyaluronidase, which exists in the bee venom. Its function in the venom is to break down mammalian tissue and allow the other toxins in the venom to diffuse deeper into the wound. This enzyme is also found in certain bacteria and in snake venom. But it is interesting that it is also present in malignant cancer cells where again its function is to assist these cells in spreading to other areas of the body. As beekeepers are frequently exposed to hyaluronidase they will build up antibodies against it and this could help in their defence against malignant cancers and so give them time for their body's immune system to destroy them.

These are just two theories as to how one may account for the lower incidence of cancer amongst beekeepers and I am sure one could think of others, or I suppose, even dismiss the whole idea.

But before one goes so far as to do this, let us look at the possibility of honey being the explanation. Not that one would seriously consider honey to have any effect on transformed cells, but could honey have another significant role in the prevention of cancer?

In recent years it has become generally recognised that incorrect diet is a major cause of cancer in man. Cooked food, for example, particularly that containing burnt, or browned material derived during its heating, is particularly pin-pointed to be a likely cause. This has been confirmed by feeding this browned material to experimental rodents when it was found to cause cancers in the majority of instances. In addition the browning reaction products formed during the caramelization of sugars or on their reaction with amino acids when heated are also known to be carcinogenic.

Although some mass-produced honey would contain these substances, home-produced honey is completely free of them. One can easily prove this by taking a small amount of a commercial honey and mixing it with an equal volume of water. If this is allowed to stand in a wine glass overnight, one will find next morning a dirty deposit of material at the bottom of the glass. No such material forms if the honey is home-produced. One would conclude from this that eating pure honey must have an advantage over other varieties. It is pertinent to point out that the honey recommended by Galen and other figures from antiquity was described as 'raw' honey, meaning, of course, unprocessed honey.

Honey described in this way not only would be unheated honey, but would be mainly comb honey. Comb honey also might have a significant role in preventing cancer. Could not the consumption of large amounts of the beeswax present in the honeycomb act in a similar manner to eating fibre? Today, eating adequate fibre is widely accepted as being a dietary habit that significantly reduces the possibility of certain cancers.

Although some of the above remarks remain in the realm of speculation, they nevertheless have some scientific foundation. It would be foolish to think that eating honey alone will solve everyone's health problems as clearly there are many factors involved. For one thing, anyone who is sensible enough to go out of their way to make sure they are eating genuine pure unprocessed honey is also going to do the same thing with other foods. So it could be one's overall general attitude to food, rather than any particular item. What we can say conclusively is, eating pure honey may, at best, do tremendous good and, at least, have no particular benefit. One thing we can be absolutely certain about is, it can do no harm, and there are a few foods that that can said about!

CHAPTER 13

Natural or Unnatural Medicine?

Alternative medicine is on the increase in Britain today, so much so, that the British Medical Association has recently set up an inquiry to study what role it might have in modern medical practice. What seems to have disturbed the BMA most is not so much the increasing number of patients flocking to various forms of alternative treatment but the significant number of their own membership who are adopting these scientifically discarded methods. In one of their recent surveys it was found that around 300 doctors are now practising homoeopathy, and many others are resorting to such procedures as acupuncture and hypnosis. What has been the cause for this reversal in what was previously an aspiring trend in the progress of medical science?

One of the root causes, I believe, is the motivation of the pharmaceutical companies. These commercial concerns now wield tremendous influence over modern medical practice. They exist, however, not for the prime function of improving people's health, but for making money. Because of this much of the philosophical basis of today's chemotherapy is questionable. It would be foolish to go to the extreme, as some have done, and pronounce that all drugs should be banned and we return to herbs. Far from it, for many of the drugs available today play a crucial role, but, on the other hand, many drugs prescribed today are unnecessary, and those that are useful are often grossly misused.

The philosophy that takes for granted that there is a 'pill for every ill' has its origins in the operational approach adopted by the drug industry. Firstly, at a scientific level they influence the direction of research. Many of the major medical journals, for example, are dependent upon funding received directly from the pharmaceutical industry. Under these circumstances, what medical journal is going to promulgate the views of natural medicine? Consequently natural medicines tend to be condemned outright. Furthermore, they influence the type of research carried out by directly sponsoring university research, and by supporting selected scientific meetings, thereby encouraging research into particular areas that might be useful to themselves. If they were really interested in the health of people they would fund research into areas unlikely to lead to patentable products, such as natural medicines. This they fail to do.

Their greatest influence, however, is directly with the doctors themselves. A recent survey of the medical profession has revealed that particular drugs are prescribed by doctors mainly under influence from the pharmaceutical companies. In 1982, for example, the industry spent £150 million on drug promotion in Britain. This works out at around £5000 for every general practitioner. It is estimated that there is now one drug company representative for every eight doctors.

Is it any wonder that this kind of medicine has, in many people's eyes, been seen to be a failure, and that the type of medical care received today is in some ways inferior to that of a generation ago.

Drift from Science

I believe that there is a much deeper cause for the drift away from scientific medicine, and this is a consequence of the failure of the scientific revolution. In the years immediately following World War II science was heralded as the means by which the New Jerusalem was to be built. Today, however, this vision has become rather tarnished. The euphoria that followed the introduction of antibiotics quickly faded in the wake of the thalidomide scandal. The cheap electricity that was promised by the nuclear industry is now seen to have been bought at a price, paid for in pollution of the environment. Awareness, resulting from Chernobyl, the Three Mile Island accident in the United States, and the emergence of the true facts of the 1957 Windscale accident, have made people less prepared to accept these so-called advances at their face value.

Although modern agriculture has thrived by widespread application of more and more powerful insecticides and pesticides, the full consequences of this approach are only now becoming apparent. The accidents at Bhopal and Seveso have highlighted the true price for which scientific advances are made. Not that it is science itself that is responsible, but man, in the way he fumbles around trying to find how best to control it.

Disillusionment with Modern Medicine

When it comes to medical care, most doctors will readily admit that much of the ill-health in our society is a result of how people live and adapt to both their problems and the environment. The adoption of a philosophy that all these ills may be alleviated by means of drugs is both naive and destructive. No drug can ever be thought of as 'safe'. They all have some adverse side effects, for the so-called 'magic bullet' belongs only to medical mythology.

The upshot has been nothing other than ironic. Doctors are now seeing patients with complaints that they know will clear up on their own, without the intervention of drugs, but it is the patient who now demands and expects drug treatment. Doctors are therefore increasingly prescribing placebos, which can be seen as nothing other than a return to a form of witch-doctoring.

The more concerned members of the population see quite clearly what has happened and are leading a return to alternative forms of treatment. (However, to call these methods 'alternative' seems to me rather inappropriate, for today's 'alternative' medicine was yesterday's acceptable medicine!)

Value of Traditional Medicine

We tend to believe that because we have a greater understanding of the world about us, we therefore are somehow more intellectually competent than our forebears. In fact the opposite is probably true. Many of our ancestors were forced by necessity to develop natural treatments for diseases that were tried and tested in an empirical way over many generations. The ones to survive this rigorous test were passed on from mother to child. There was no ulterior motivation in this process other than the preservation of one's own offspring, which is the most powerful of human instincts. This type of process is far more effective than any controlled clinical trial that could be devised today.

We fail to recognise that most of our major medical advances did not arise out of the blue, but had their origins in some form of traditional medicine. Thus it was a humble milkmaid who informed Jenner about her natural cure for smallpox, which led to the development of the present science of immunology. Penicillin itself was not entirely new to medicine, for in the form of its parent mould it had been used for generations in folk medicine. Vitamin A, present in raw liver, was used by the ancient Egyptians to treat night blindness, long before its significance was recognized by modern science. The ancient Greeks used the phenols in wine to sterilize wounds long before Lister, and so one could go on. In all these traditional treatments there is now known to be a scientific basis. Thus I believe we should treat traditional medicine much more seriously than we do at present. In particular we should attempt to unravel the scientific basis of any particular remedy. This is the approach I have adopted in this book in dealing with the role of honey as a natural medicine. In fact there can be no greater tradition associated with any particular folk remedy than there exists with honey. For medical men have, from the earliest of times, made the study of bees the theme of many writings. Indeed, if one reads the writings of the ancients one will discover that there were few ills that were not curable by either honey, or some other product of bees. Can we really afford to disregard the tremendous historical association between honey and health?

Appendix

Recent Demonstrations of the Antibiotic Properties of Honey

Date	***Researchers***	***Institute***	***Country***
1978	M. Wootton, R. A. Edwards, A. Rowse	University of New South Wales	Australia
1973	N. N. Sedova, M. F. Usmanov	Academy of Medical Sciences, Moscow	USSR
1970	D. G. Steyn	University of Pretoria	South Africa
1969	M. R. Smith, W. F. McCaughey, A. R. Kemmerer	University of Arizona	USA
1968	W. Mohrig, B. Messner	Ernst-Moritz-Arndt University, Greifswald	DDR
1966	M. Chwastek	Sanitarno Epidermiologiczna Stacja Bydgoszcz	Poland
1966	R. Buchner	Freibrug	W. Germany
1966	J. P. Chambonnaud	Apicultural Research Laboratory, Nice	France
1963	M. R. Smith	University of Arizona	USA

1963	P. Lavie	Laboratory of Experimental Apiculture, Montfavet	France
1962	K. Rizvanov, B. Bizhev	Inst. of Agriculture, Sofia	Bulgaria
1962	K. E. Lindner	Karl Marx University, Liepzig	DDR
1961	G. Khristov & S. Mladenov	Vissh Medical Institute, Sofia	Bulgaria
1961	A. d'Agostino-Barbaro, C. La Rosa, C. Zannelli	University of Messina, Sicily	Italy
1960	J. Stomfay-Stitz & S. D. Kominos	Dept. of Biology, Duquesne University, Pittsburgh	USA
1956	R. Schuler & R. Vogel	University of München	W. Germany
1955	H. Dold, R. Witzenhausen	University of Freiburg	W. Germany
1954	G. P. Brangi, M. Pavan	University of Pavia	Italy
1950	F. J. Pothman	Institute of Medicine, Dusseldorf	W. Germany

Index

Royal Jelly

A Guide To Nature's Richest Health Food

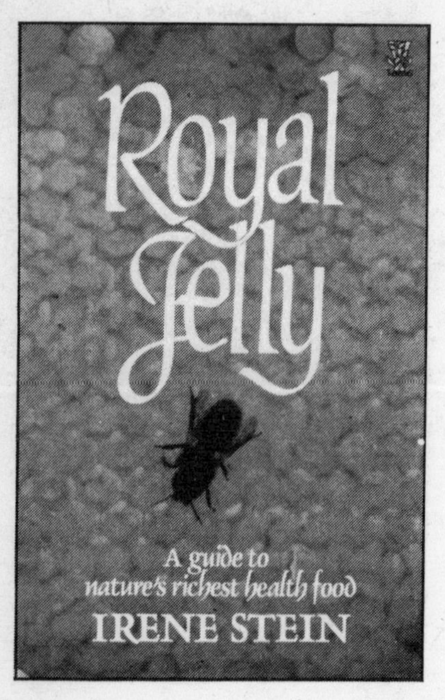

The food of Queen's — queen bees to be specific. Specially produced by bees, this super food is capable of turning a perfectly ordinary chrysalis into that magnificent specimen — the Queen Bee. **Irene Stein,** a health and beauty expert, has been actively involved in research into Royal Jelly for over twelve years. In this easy-to-read volume she explains the many health-giving properties of this unique food including: increased alertness; calmness and efficiency; tip-top bodily fitness; shining hair; glowing complexion; strong nails and increased resistance to disease. Used regularly by such celebrities as Sebastian Coe, Cliff Richard, Joe Brown and Barbara Cartland, this remarkable substance really IS nature's richest food.